FAST FACTS ABOUT EKGs FOR NURSES

Michele Angell Landrum, ADN, RN, CCRN, is a clinical nurse educator with the Staff Development Department at Springhill Medical Center in Mobile, Alabama, where she teaches the RN EKG training program and AHA ACLS and PALS courses. She also assisted in the development of EKG courses for monitor technicians who have no prior medical/cardiac training. Michele received her associate degree in nursing from the University of Mobile in 1998 and is actively pursuing her bachelor's degree in nursing at Jacksonville University. She has worked in various facilities throughout the United States, such as North Shore University Hospital–LIJ in Manhasset, New York, and Cedars-Sinai Hospital in Los Angeles. Her specialties include the cardiac care unit, cardiovascular intensive care unit, surgical intensive care unit, emergency room, cardiac catheterization lab, and electrophysiology lab. She has authored two books for Springer Publishing Company: *Fast Facts for the Travel Nurse* (2010) and *Fast Facts for the Critical Care Nurse* (2012).

FAST FACTS ABOUT EKGs FOR NURSES

Michele Angell Landrum, ADN, RN, CCRN, is a clinical nurse educator with the Staff Development Department at Springhill Medical Center in Mobile, Alabama, where she teaches the RN EKG training program and AHA ACLS and PALS courses. She also assisted in the development of EKG courses for monitor technicians who have no prior medical/cardiac training. Michele received her associate degree in nursing from the University of Mobile in 1998 and is actively pursuing her bachelor's degree in nursing at Jacksonville University. She has worked in various facilities throughout the United States, such as North Shore University Hospital–LIJ in Manhasset, New York, and Cedars-Sinai Hospital in Los Angeles. Her specialties include the cardiac care unit, cardiovascular intensive care unit, surgical intensive care unit, emergency room, cardiac catheterization lab, and electrophysiology lab. She has authored two books for Springer Publishing Company: *Fast Facts for the Travel Nurse* (2010) and *Fast Facts for the Critical Care Nurse* (2012).

FAST FACTS ABOUT EKGs FOR NURSES

The Rules of Identifying EKGs in a Nutshell

Michele Angell Landrum, ADN, RN, CCRN

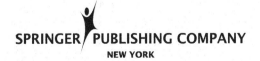

SPRINGER PUBLISHING COMPANY

NEW YORK

Springer Publishing Company, LLC
11 West 42nd Street
New York, NY 10036
www.springerpub.com

Acquisitions Editor: Margaret Zuccarini
Composition: S4Carlisle Publishing Services

ISBN: 978-0-8261-2006-9
e-book ISBN: 978-0-8261-2007-6

13 14 15 16 17 / 5 4 3 2 1

The author and the publisher of this Work have made every effort to use sources believed to be reliable to provide information that is accurate and compatible with the standards generally accepted at the time of publication. Because medical science is continually advancing, our knowledge base continues to expand. Therefore, as new information becomes available, changes in procedures become necessary. We recommend that the reader always consult current research and specific institutional policies before performing any clinical procedure. The author and publisher shall not be liable for any special, consequential, or exemplary damages resulting, in whole or in part, from the readers' use of, or reliance on, the information contained in this book. The publisher has no responsibility for the persistence or accuracy of URLs for external or third-party Internet websites referred to in this publication and does not guarantee that any content on such websites is, or will remain, accurate or appropriate.

Library of Congress Cataloging-in-Publication Data
Landrum, Michele Angell.
  Fast facts about EKGs for nurses : the rules of identifying EKGs in a nutshell / Michele Angell Landrum.
    p. ; cm.
  Includes bibliographical references and index.
  ISBN 978-0-8261-2006-9 — ISBN 0-8261-2006-7 — ISBN 978-0-8261-2007-6 (e-book)
  I. Title.
  [DNLM: 1. Electrocardiography—methods—Nurses' Instruction. 2. Arrhythmias, Cardiac—diagnosis—Nurses' Instruction. WG 140]
  RC683.5.E5
  616.1'207547—dc23   2013015356

Printed in the United States of America by Gasch Printing.

This book is dedicated to my sons, Carter and Cody, for it is their love that makes every day a blessing.

—M.A.L.

Contents

Preface

Nursing is a complex and challenging career. The joy and pain encountered in this fascinating, dynamic profession are rewarding and constant. Learning is not finished when one graduates from a university, but continues throughout one's lifetime. The reasons for continued learning are varied, ranging from changes in technology and the health care system to a change in practice venue.

Understanding the electrical function of the human heart and the ability to identify EKG rhythm strips are valuable skills to both new and senior nurses. This knowledge is paramount when caring for patients in medical facilities and is also important when reviewing charts for court, case management, and/or quality control. Nurses practicing in clinics, on ambulances, and in various locations within the armed services will also benefit from these skills. Being able to identify EKG rhythms with confidence is an excellent attribute for anyone in the nursing field.

Fast Facts About EKGs for Nurses provides the foundation for understanding the electrical function of the heart. The simplest terms are used and a "box" diagram is the basis for describing the electrical conduction system. After just the first few chapters, a crystal-clear comprehension of this system and its components dawns.

Once the functional foundation is laid, a detailed step-by-step approach to deciphering the actual EKG rhythm strip and its components is explained. This method has been taught multiple times to nurses practicing in and out of the hospital setting with varying experience levels—from new graduate to 20-plus-year veterans—and the outcome is always the same. They get it! Frequent comments upon course completion include "I wish I had taken this class sooner!" and "I really didn't understand EKG strips at all and now I feel great about them." The technique is simple and easy to follow.

After the mastery of rhythm strip complexes and identification techniques, the most widely documented EKG rhythms are discussed in detail. There are actual EKG strip examples of each rhythm. Practice strips and scenarios are included in this manual.

This book can serve as a self-learning experience, a refresher course, and/or the basis for an EKG class. It is an incredible tool for new and experienced nurses alike.

Please keep in mind that this manual was developed using numerous resources combined with multiple years of cardiac nursing experience. The techniques and scenarios detailed are useful and very real. However, it is important to follow American Heart Association and facility protocols along with physician's orders. Personal and patient safety is always of primary concern.

Michele Angell Landrum, ADN, RN, CCRN

Acknowledgments

Thank you to all the wonderful nurses and staff with whom I have had the joy to work and teach the last few years. It is through education, preceptorship, training, and teamwork that I was able to develop the skills required for EKG identification and the ability to share the technique with others. I have learned so much from my students and appreciate their efforts to master this difficult subject.

Much appreciation goes to Jane Davis, MS, Scott Wilson, BA, RN, Catherine Hundley, BSN, RN, Ginny Bennett, BS, and Stephanie Darst, BA, for their support and encouragement.

As always, special thanks to my family and friends. You all have been so incredibly patient, supportive, and understanding. Each of you means more to me than you will ever know.

Finally, thank you to my husband and sons, Ted, Carter, and Cody. The joy and unconditional love you three give are remarkable.

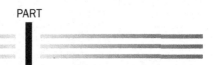

Understanding the Basics of EKGs

1

Basic Cardiac Anatomy

Prior to the evaluation of an EKG strip, the cardiac anatomy, the mechanical function of the heart, and the heart's electrical conduction must be understood. This chapter explains cardiac anatomy in its simplest terms. Do not let the anatomy of the heart be intimidating. It will be demystified in the following pages. Electrical conduction is discussed in Chapter 2.

In this chapter, you will learn:

1. Basic cardiac anatomy
2. Basic cardiac mechanical function

KEY CARDIAC FACTS

Every nurse knows the heart. Key facts serve as a reminder of cardiac function, location, and importance. The terms are simple and easy to understand.

==*FAST FACTS in a NUTSHELL*

1. The heart is a hollow muscular organ that pumps blood through the body.
2. The heart is about the size of the human fist.
3. The heart weighs approximately 10.5 ounces.
4. The heart pumps 4 to 8 liters of blood per minute.
5. The heart of an average adult beats 70 times per minute.
6. The heart is located posterior to the sternum and anterior to the spine, resting between the lungs, superior to the diaphragm.
7. The heart is composed of three layers: the epicardium, the myocardium, and the endocardium, the innermost layer.
8. The heart has four chambers: two atria and two ventricles.
9. The heart has four one-way valves: tricuspid, mitral, pulmonic, and aortic.
10. The heart has a septum that divides it into a right and left side.
11. Coronary arteries are located on the epicardium and supply the myocardium with blood.

BASIC CARDIAC ANATOMY

The heart can be explained in several ways with numerous descriptions and "characterizations." However, the simplest way is to picture it as a box. This particular box has four divisions inside and a few tubes coming out. See Figure 1.1.

The divisions can be labeled with the common cardiac terms: right atrium, left atrium, right ventricle, and left ventricle. The tubes can be labeled with the terms: superior vena cava, pulmonary artery, pulmonary veins, and aorta. See Figure 1.2, which depicts the "box" with its corresponding labels.

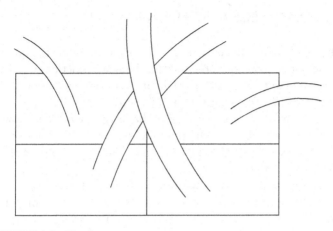

FIGURE 1.1 The heart.

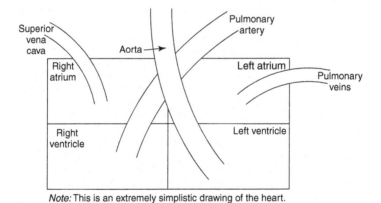

Note: This is an extremely simplistic drawing of the heart.

FIGURE 1.2 The heart as a "box."

FAST FACTS in a NUTSHELL

The heart can easily be depicted as a "box" that has multiple functions.

CARDIAC MECHANICAL FUNCTION

The heart's job is to circulate blood. This is accomplished with muscular contractions creating "mechanical" function. Unoxygenated blood flows into the right atrium via the superior vena cava and then flows into the right ventricle. It is then pushed into the lungs to receive oxygen. The oxygenated blood flows into the left atrium via the pulmonary veins. The blood then travels down to the left ventricle, which pumps the oxygen-rich blood to the body.

The sequence occurs with every heartbeat, leading to an average of 6 liters of blood pumped per minute. This muscular contraction is caused by the heart's electrical conduction system.

2

Cardiac Electrical Conduction

The heart's electrical conduction system can be just as confusing and as hard to understand as cardiac anatomy. This chapter provides an explanation of the system in easy-to-understand terms. It simplifies the knowledge of cardiac electrical conduction required to properly identify EKG rhythms.

In this chapter, you will learn:

1. The electrical components of the heart
2. The conduction pathway of the heart
3. How myocardial cell depolarization and repolarization occur

THE COMPONENTS OF CARDIAC ELECTRICAL CONDUCTION

The heart is composed of myocardial cells. These specialized cells allow electrical impulses to travel through cardiac tissue. All myocardial cells possess three characteristics: automaticity, conductivity, and contractility. This uniqueness gives each cell in the heart the ability to initiate an electrical impulse, to transfer or "conduct" an electrical impulse, and to contract. While every cell in the heart has these capabilities, certain components align to form a "conduction pathway" that helps the heart to work efficiently.

It is very important to remember that electrical activity in the heart does not always lead to mechanical activity. An unhealthy heart cannot always contract as efficiently as the electrical impulses indicate. A heart in cardiac tamponade, for example, may not contract at all.

=FAST FACTS in a NUTSHELL

The major components of cardiac electrical conduction pathway are:

1. The sinus (SA) node
2. The AV node
3. The bundle of His
4. The bundle branches
5. The Purkinje fibers

THE CONDUCTION PATHWAY OF THE HEART

Electrical conduction within the heart occurs via polarization of the myocardial cells. It can occur cell to cell but works most effectively when the electrical conduction pathway is followed with each heartbeat. Each area of the conduction pathway consists of myocardial cells that are specific to their location. See Figure 2.1 for a diagram depicting the normal conduction pathway.

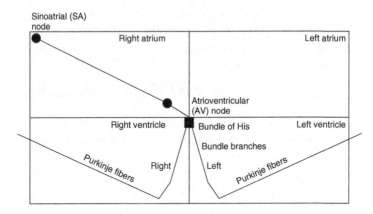

FIGURE 2.1   The normal cardiac conduction pathway.

The conduction pathway starts in the high right atrium with the sinoatrial node, frequently referred to as the SA node. This is the location where most heartbeats originate and is often known as the "pacemaker" of the heart. The SA node has an intrinsic rate of 60 to 100 impulses per minute.

After the SA node initiates an electrical impulse, it travels down the right atrium along the conduction pathway to the atrioventricular node, better known as the AV node. This area is located at the "junction" of the right atrium and right ventricle near the septal wall between the atrium. This area will slow the impulse slightly to allow blood to flow from the atria to the ventricles. The AV node has an intrinsic rate of 40 to 60 impulses per minute and could take over as the "pacemaker" of the heart if the SA node fails.

Next, the impulse travels to the bundle of His, located just below the AV node in the septum of the heart near the top of the ventricles. Following the bundle of His in the conduction pathway are the bundle branches. They are located along the septum of the ventricles and run parallel in separate right and left sides or "branches."

Finally, the electrical impulse reaches the Purkinje fibers. These finger-like projections are woven into the dense, fibrous, ventricular tissue. The intrinsic rate of the ventricles is 20 to 40 impulses per minute.

===*FAST FACTS in a NUTSHELL*

The conduction of one electrical impulse through the heart is considered the completion of one cardiac cycle.

As already explained, the AV node possesses the ability to take over as the "pacemaker" of the heart if the SA node fails. The ventricles could also take over if both of the higher pathway components fail. However, the rate would be very slow. The ventricles do not make a stable site for impulse initiation because ventricular "pacemaker" sites fail quickly. The failure of conduction pathway components can be caused by various medical issues such as myocardial cell death, scarring, electrolyte problems, and/or drug toxicities.

While the heart possesses a fail-safe system for cardiac conduction, the following fact is also true: Whichever area of the heart is initiating impulses the fastest can become the pacemaker, or "driver," of the heart. For example, if a super-excited area in the ventricle begins to conduct electrical impulses at a rate of 300 beats per minute, the resulting rhythm would be ventricular tachycardia. This occurs because the rate of the ventricular area exceeds the rate of the SA node. This will be further explained in later chapters.

===*FAST FACTS in a NUTSHELL*

The intrinsic rate of the conduction pathway components:

SA node = 60–100 impulses per minute
AV node = 40–60 impulses per minute
Ventricles = 20–40 impulses per minute

MYOCARDIAL CELL POLARIZATION

The ability to initiate and conduct an electrical impulse in an attempt to cause muscular contraction is facilitated by myocardial cell depolarization and repolarization. A basic understanding of this cycle is required to properly identify EKGs.

Polarization is "technically" the resting state of a cardiac cell during which no electrical activity occurs in the heart (www.nuclearcardiologyseminars.net/electrophysiology .htm). The cell is negatively charged.

Depolarization happens when the movement of ions across the cell membrane causes the cell to become more positive. During atrial depolarization, the atria should be contracting to push blood through the valves into the ventricles. During ventricular depolarization, the ventricles should be contracting, forcing blood out to the body and lungs. Depolarization is the "doing" phase of cardiac tissue.

Repolarization occurs when the movement of ions across the cell membrane causes the cell to return to a negative charge. During repolarization, the muscular tissue should be resting. The atrium and ventricles "relax" during repolarization.

Myocardial cell depolarization and repolarization correspond with the EKG rhythm. When a P wave is seen, the atria are depolarizing. During the QRS, the atria are repolarizing and the ventricles are depolarizing. The T wave is illustrative of the ventricles repolarizing. This will be further explained in chapters to come.

═══════════════════════════════════*FAST FACTS in a NUTSHELL*

- Atrial depolarization is signified by the P wave on an EKG strip.
- Ventricular depolarization is signified by the QRS complex on an EKG strip.
- Ventricular repolarization is signified by the T wave on an EKG strip.

3

The Cardiac Cycle and the Rhythm Strip

The cardiac cycle and the rhythm strip go hand in hand. A healthy heart functions in an extremely repetitive pattern that can be displayed on paper. This tracing is called a rhythm, or EKG, strip. The strip can be broken down into several key pieces that, when properly identified, provide insight into the heart's function and health.

In this chapter, you will learn:

1. The components of the cardiac cycle
2. The proper sequence of the cardiac cycle
3. The components of a rhythm (EKG) strip
4. The appearance of the rhythm strip of a healthy heart

THE CARDIAC CYCLE

The cardiac cycle is most simply described as one heartbeat. It should produce the rhythmic contraction of the cardiac muscle, including systole and diastole.

The beginning of the cardiac cycle is the depolarization of the SA node and the end is the repolarization of ventricles.

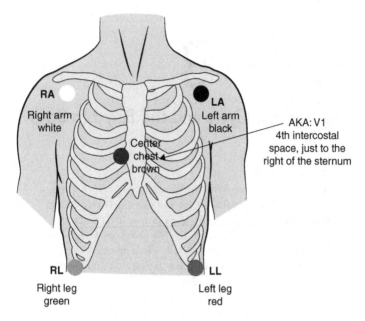

FIGURE 3.1   5-lead EKG electrode placement.

These events can be depicted on paper via electrodes attached to the exterior chest wall of a patient (Figure 3.1). The electrodes are connected to cables and the cables are then coupled to a module where the information is translated into the EKG rhythm strip.

Each component of the EKG rhythm strip corresponds to the electrical events of the cardiac cycle as depicted in Figure 3.2.

THE RHYTHM STRIP

When looking at a rhythm strip (EKG 3.1), a clinician initially focuses on single beat, or cardiac cycle. There are three major components to consider: the P wave, the QRS complex, and the T wave.

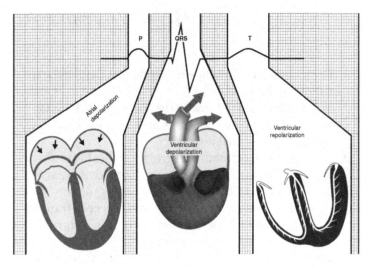

FIGURE 3.2 EKG strip components in correlation to the cardiac cycle.

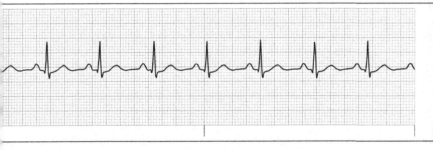

EKG 3.1 EKG strip of a sinus rhythm.

The P wave corresponds to the atria depolarizing and is indicative of atrial contraction. The QRS complex corresponds with depolarization of the ventricles, indicating ventricular contraction. The T wave corresponds to the ventricular repolarization during which the heart is preparing for another contraction.

=== *FAST FACTS in a NUTSHELL*

Key Points to Remember:

- The tracing on a rhythm strip represents the electrical activity of the heart only!
- In a normal healthy heart, the mechanical function occurs as stated; however, this may not be the case in unhealthy, abnormal hearts.
- The electrical activity occurring in the heart that is producing the highest current (output) is what is visualized on the EKG strip. This is why there is not an electrical tracing signifying atrial repolarization (resting). This activity occurs while the ventricles are depolarizing (working/doing), which produces much more electrical current (output) than atrial repolarization.

4

The Rhythm Strip

The rhythm (EKG) strip is the basis for identifying an EKG rhythm. A general understanding of the strip and its components is required to identify cardiac rhythms. Basic information regarding the waveforms representing the cardiac cycle and the rhythm strip itself is needed.

In this chapter, you will learn:

1. How to navigate a rhythm strip
2. The normal measurements of the rhythm strip components
3. How to calculate the rate of a rhythm strip

THE PAPER AND ITS BOXES

The paper a rhythm strip is printed on is generally standard throughout the world. It is a small piece of graph-type paper, most often printed in black ink. The "graph" boxes may be red or black. There may be 1-, 3-, or 5-lead readings displayed on the paper. See EKG 4.1 for an example of a rhythm strip.

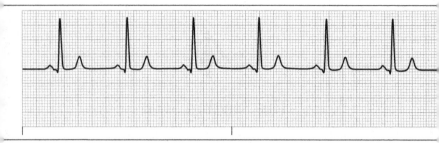

EKG 4.1   Rhythm strip of sinus rhythm.

In this book, all examples will exhibit a rhythm in a single lead (lead II). All will be printed on black graph boxes with the EKG tracing also in black.

The EKG paper is covered entirely in boxes. These boxes are extremely important. They are paramount in identifying an EKG rhythm and its components.

The boxes on EKG paper represent time. A rhythm strip is read, or "studied," from left to right when discussing time. Each small box measures 0.04 seconds. Each large box, depicted by the darker, bolder lines, contains five small boxes and measures 0.20 seconds of time (Figure 4.1).

These box measurements, coupled with the three black marks along the top or bottom of the rhythm strip, allow EKG rhythm identification to be performed.

EKG strips can also be measured in amplitude. How tall a particular EKG component is corresponds to its amplitude, but this measurement is not required for basic EKG identification. It gains importance as 12-lead EKG evaluation is performed. The "height," or amplitude, is observed as how far away the complex is from the iso-electric line, or "baseline," of the strip (see EKG 4.4).

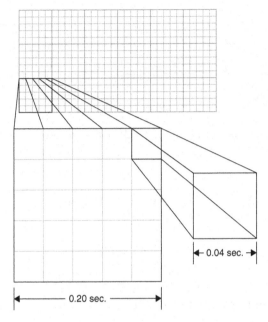

FIGURE 4.1   EKG paper with a close-up of small and large boxes.

===*FAST FACTS in a NUTSHELL*

The three black marks across the top (EKG 4.2) or bottom (EKG 4.3) of the strip indicate 6 seconds of time.

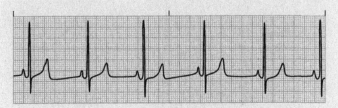

EKG 4.2   Strip with top tick marks representing 6 seconds of time.

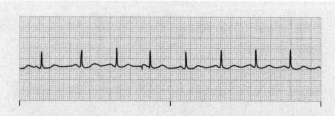

EKG 4.3 Strip with bottom tick marks representing 6 seconds of time.

THE CARDIAC CYCLE COMPONENTS OF THE RHYTHM STRIP

The waves depicted on the EKG strip correspond to electrical activity in the heart. The cardiac cycle is thus represented as well. Each wave has set values that correlate with the amount of time it takes healthy cardiac tissue to perform the activity it represents.

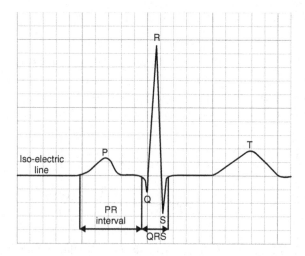

EKG 4.4 Normal EKG strip with wave measurements depicting where to begin and stop measuring and noting iso-electric line.

The P wave is not measured alone. When referring to its measurement, the area from where the P wave leaves the iso-electric line until the beginning of QRS complex is taken into account. This is called the PR interval, or PRI. The normal distance of the PRI is between 0.12 and 0.20 seconds.

A normal QRS measures between 0.04 and 0.10 seconds. It is measured from where the QRS complex leaves the iso-electric line to when it returns to the iso-electric line. The QRS complex may not always contain a Q wave, an R wave, and an S wave, but it is still considered the QRS complex. (There are some schools of thought that allow the QRS to measure up to 0.12 seconds and still be considered normal. As of the publication date of this book, the generalized standard remains 0.04 to 0.10 seconds but could increase to 0.12 seconds as medical knowledge advances.)

The QT length can be measured, and normal is 0.35 to 0.44 seconds. However, this is not a major focus in basic EKG identification. The QT interval can be affected by heart rate and is often influenced by medications. The T wave is not routinely measured in regard to duration of time in basic EKG identification.

═══════════════════════════*FAST FACTS in a NUTSHELL*

- EKG 4.4 is one of the most important EKGs in this manual, as it is the basis for all rhythm strip identification.
- Remember to read EKG strips from left to right.
- When measuring component intervals, do not count the starting line the complex directly falls on. Begin counting with the first line moving forward from left to right.

Other measurements can be obtained from a rhythm strip, such as ST segment elevation. However, this is not required for basic EKG rhythm identification.

RHYTHM STRIP RATE CALCULATION

There are two methods to calculate the rate of an EKG strip. The easiest way to determine the rate of a rhythm strip is as follows:

1. Acquire a 6-second strip. This is a strip that has the three tick marks on it (see EKG 4.2 and EKG 4.3).
2. Identify the QRS.
3. Count the number of R waves in the 6-second strip. Do not count pre-ventricular contractions (PVCs) in rate determination. (See Chapter 9 for detailed information regarding PVCs.)
4. Multiply the number of R waves by 10.

   The result is the rate of the strip, which is also the patient's heart rate and the ventricular rate. See EKG 4.5 for an example.

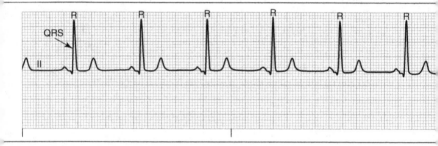

EKG 4.5 Sinus rhythm with rate calculation illustrated. These steps are taken to calculate the rate for this strip. 1. Three tick marks on the bottom (30 big boxes) denote a 6-second strip. 2. Identify the QRS complexes. 3. Six R waves are noted on this strip. 4. 6 × 10 = 60. The ventricular rate of this strip is 60.

Following are several practice EKG strips. Calculate the rate and measure the intervals. Do not attempt rhythm identification at this time. The answers follow the examples. Unless otherwise noted, all rhythm strips in this manual are 6 seconds of time.

PRACTICE RATE CALCULATION
AND INTERVAL MEASUREMENT STRIPS

1.

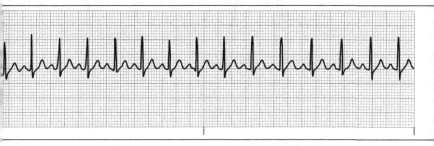

    Rate:

    PRI:

    QRS:

2.

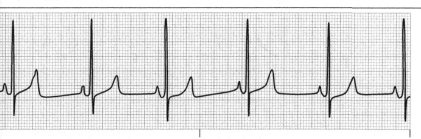

    Rate:

    PRI:

    QRS:

3.

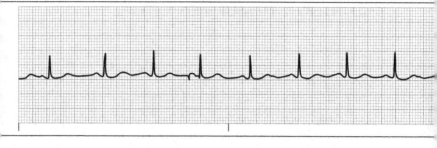

Rate:

PRI:

QRS:

4.

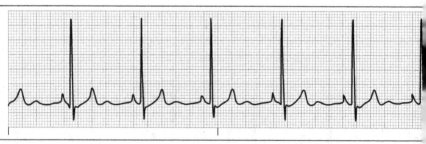

Rate:

PRI:

QRS:

5.

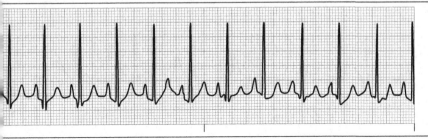

Rate:

PRI:

QRS:

6.

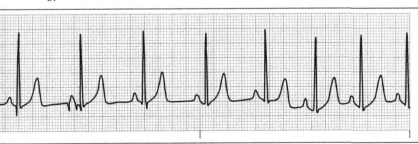

Rate:

PRI:

QRS:

7.

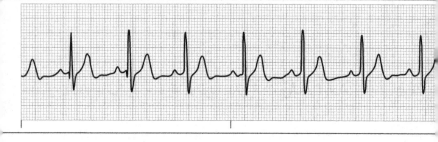

Rate:

PRI:

QRS:

8.

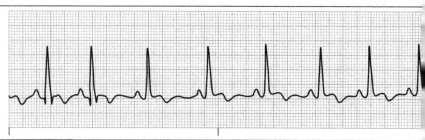

Rate:

PRI:

QRS:

9.

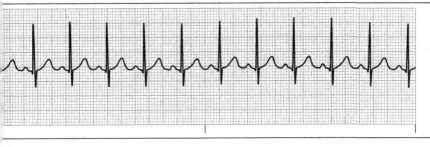

Rate:

PRI:

QRS:

10.

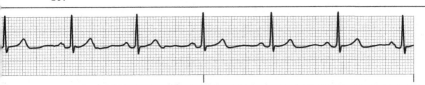

Rate:

PRI:

QRS:

ANSWERS TO RATE CALCULATION AND INTERVAL MEASUREMENT STRIPS

Note: When identifying EKG strip component measurements, it is acceptable to be within 0.02- to 0.03-second difference from the answers. This is related to the complex nature of the electrical system of the heart. The measurements may vary minutely from beat to beat. However, this variance should not change the overall identification of the strip. For example, if the PRI answer is 0.16, the acceptable range for answers would be 0.14 to 0.18. There is also the possibility that a component may take up one half of the small box. For example, the QRS may measure 0.06 seconds. The rate calculation answer has no variance; that is, a rate of 60 is the rate of 60.

1. Rate: 150
   PRI: 0.16
   QRS: 0.08

2. Rate: 60
   PRI: 0.12
   QRS: 0.04

3. Rate: 80
   PRI: 0.16
   QRS: 0.04

4. Rate: 60
   PRI: 0.12
   QRS: 0.06

5. Rate: 120
   PRI: 0.12
   QRS: 0.04

6. Rate: 80
   PRI: 0.12
   QRS: 0.04

7. Rate: 70
   PRI: 0.16
   QRS: 0.10

8. Rate: 80
   PRI: 0.12
   QRS: 0.08

9. Rate: 120
   PRI: 0.12
   QRS: 0.08

10. Rate: 70
    PRI: 0.16
    QRS: 0.08

5

"Reading" the EKG

Reading an EKG is also known as identifying the rhythm. It is often referred to as "putting it all together" in EKG classes. It is easily completed in just a few steps, the first being rate calculation. Waveform measurement is second, and rhythm identification is performed after strip analysis. Each step is detailed in this chapter.

In this chapter, you will learn:

1. The step-by-step process of measuring a rhythm strip
2. How to determine if the strip is abnormal

THE MEASURING PROCESS

A step-by-step approach works best for EKG rhythm identification. Once analysis is complete, the rhythm can be identified as normal or abnormal. If abnormal, the measurements will be used to determine the identity of the rhythm strip.

---

1. What is the rate?
2. Is the rhythm regular?
3. Are there P waves?
4. What is the PR interval?
5. Is the QRS normal?

Other factors to consider fall under these five main steps.

EXHIBIT 5.1   The basic 5-step process of measuring an EKG strip.

Refer to Exhibit 5.1 for the basic steps utilized to determine the normality of a rhythm strip.

Step 1: The first step is to determine the rate of the strip. This is done as discussed in Chapter 4. A rate of 60 to 100 is considered normal. Rates above and below this range are abnormal. Nursing interventions related to an abnormal heart rate are based on specific patient criteria.

Do not calculate PVCs (see Chapter 9) in the rate. Variances in atrial and ventricular rates are discussed in Chapter 10.

Step 2: Determine if the rate is regular. To determine regularity, observe that the R-R interval remains constant throughout the strip. An irregular R-R interval deems the strip abnormal. See EKG 5.1 for examples of a regular R-R interval that "marches out," and an irregular R-R interval that is abnormal.

Step 3: The third step involves the P wave. Several questions must be answered regarding the P wave:

1. Are there P waves in this EKG strip?
2. If yes, are they regular (EKG 5.2)?
3. Is there one P wave for every QRS?
4. If yes, does it fall before or after the QRS?
5. Is the P wave upright in lead II?
6. Is there one and only P wave for each QRS?
7. Do all the P waves look the same?

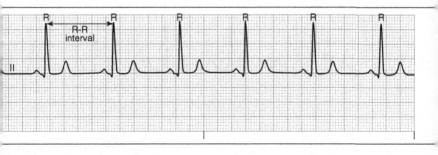

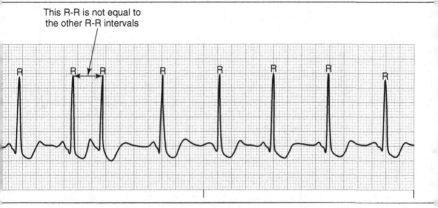

EKG 5.1   Examples of R-R regularity and irregularity. **Top**, sinus rhythm with R-R "march out." The R-R interval is generally equal throughout the strip. **Bottom**, sinus rhythm with a premature atrial contraction showing an irregular R-R interval.

When no is the answer to Questions 1 through 3 or 5 through 7, the strip is abnormal. The rhythm is also abnormal if the answer to question 4 is that the P wave falls after the QRS.

Step 4: The PR interval is measured (refer to Ch. 4). The interval must fall between 0.12 and 0.20 seconds to be considered normal. It should be constant from beat to beat. If it varies, the strip is abnormal. If PR interval variation is observed, note if there is a pattern. (Chapter 10 discusses varying PR intervals in detail.)

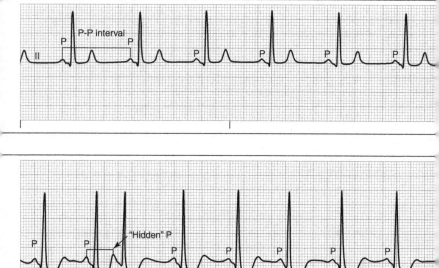

EKG 5.2 Examples of P wave regularity and irregularity. P-P regularity is determined by measuring the P-P interval in a manner similar to measuring the R-R interval. **Top,** sinus rhythm measuring regular P-P interval. **Bottom,** sinus rhythm with a premature atrial contraction showing an abnormal P-P interval.

════════════════════════════ *FAST FACTS in a NUTSHELL*

Normal measurements for an EKG strip are:

- Ventricular rate: 60 to 100
- PRI: 0.12 to 0.20 seconds
- QRS: 0.04 to 0.10 seconds

Other components are also considered to determine normality.

Step 5: Finally, in Step 5, the QRS is evaluated. It must measure between 0.04 and 0.10 (refer to Ch. 4) or it is considered abnormal. A wider QRS is either a bundle branch block or ventricular ectopy, both of which are discussed in later chapters. Each QRS in the strip should be similar in width and appearance.

Again, it is important to be aware that there is some thought in the medical community to allowing a QRS width of up to 0.12 seconds to qualify as normal. The consensus is split. At the time of this writing, 0.04 to 0.10 seconds is the gold standard for normal QRS duration. A variance of 0.02 is not of extreme significance; however, it may warrant further evaluation by a cardiologist.

If all the above criteria fall into the normal range, normal sinus rhythm is identified (EKG 5.3).

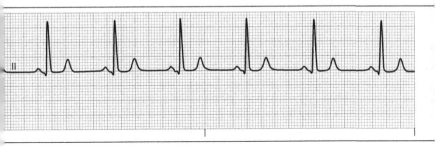

EKG 5.3   Sinus rhythm.

PART

II

Learning to Recognize the More Common Cardiac Rhythms

6

Sinus Rhythm

Sinus rhythm (SR) is one of the most important EKG rhythms to recognize. It is "normal." Approximately 98% of patients seen in the hospital will display this rhythm. It is imperative to understand what normal SR rhythm looks like. Without that, abnormality cannot be determined.

In this chapter, you will learn:

1. The determining factors for identifying SR
2. Several EKG rhythms closely related to SR

SINUS RHYTHM

SR is a normal EKG rhythm that is regular; it is sometimes referred to as NSR (normal sinus rhythm). SR, along with all rhythms termed "sinus," originates from the SA node. The characteristics of SR are listed in Exhibit 6.1.

> *Regularity*: R-R intervals are consistent throughout the EKG strip; rhythm is regular.
>
> *Rate*: Atrial and ventricular rates are equal. (The number of P waves is the same as the number of QRS complexes displayed on the EKG strip.)
>
> *Heart rate*: 60–100 beats per minute (bpm).
>
> *P wave*: All P waves in the strip have a similar, uniform appearance. There is one P wave prior to each QRS complex.
>
> *PRI*: 0.12–0.20 seconds, unchanging from beat to beat.
>
> *QRS*: 0.04–0.10 seconds.

EXHIBIT 6.1 Characteristics of sinus rhythm.

Normal SR can have various appearances. See EKGs 6.1 to 6.4.

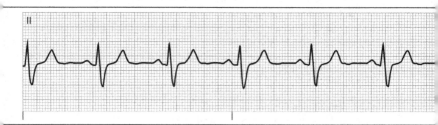

EKG 6.1 Sinus rhythm.

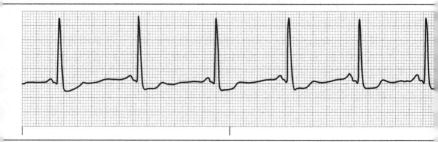

EKG 6.2 Sinus rhythm.

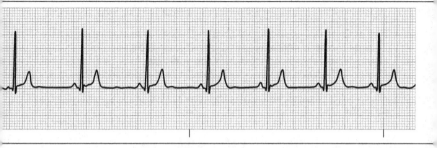

EKG 6.3 Sinus rhythm.

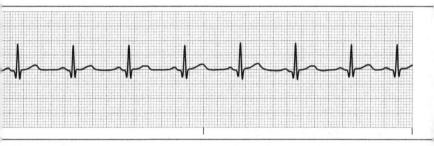

EKG 6.4 Sinus rhythm.

SINUS BRADYCARDIA

Sinus bradycardia (SB) is similar to SR. All parameters are the same except for the heart rate. See Exhibit 6.2 and EKG 6.5 for details.

Regularity: R-R intervals are consistent throughout the EKG strip, rhythm is regular.

Rate: Atrial and ventricular rates are equal. (The number of P waves is the same as the number of QRS complexes displayed on the EKG strip.)

Heart rate: Less than 60 bpm, generally above 30 bpm.

P wave: All P waves in the strip have a similar, uniform appearance. There is one P wave prior to each QRS complex.

PRI: 0.12–0.20 seconds, unchanging from beat to beat.

QRS: 0.04–0.10 seconds.

EXHIBIT 6.2 Characteristics of sinus bradycardia.

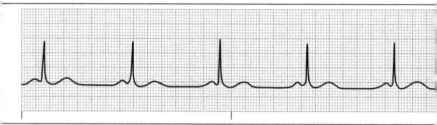

EKG 6.5 Sinus bradycardia.

There are several possible causes of SB; however, this rhythm is normal for some patients. Athletes are prone to SB due to their excellent cardiac tone while other patients exhibit SB when asleep.

Some causes of SB are the vagal response, medications (digoxin, beta blockers, etc.), chronic ischemic heart disease, and an inferior wall myocardial infarction (MI). It is important to assess each patient thoroughly and to confer with the medical team to determine if SB is "normal" or requires further investigation and possible treatment.

Treatments pertaining to SB can include atropine and dopamine infusion. Extreme symptomatic cases may require pacing.

SINUS TACHYCARDIA

Sinus tachycardia (ST) is similar to SR. All parameters are the same except the heart rate. See Exhibit 6.3 and EKG 6.6 for details.

Regularity: R-R intervals are consistent throughout the EKG strip, rhythm is regular.

Rate: Atrial and ventricular rates are equal. (The number of P waves is the same as the number of QRS complexes displayed on the EKG strip.)

Heart rate: 100–150 bpm.

P wave: All P waves in the strip have a similar, uniform appearance. There is one P wave prior to each QRS complex.

PRI: 0.12–0.20 seconds, unchanging from beat to beat.

QRS: 0.04–0.10 seconds.

EXHIBIT 6.3 Characteristics of sinus tachycardia.

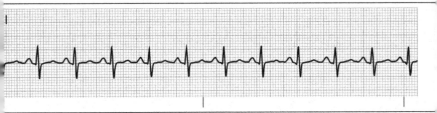

EKG 6.6 Sinus tachycardia.

There are several possible causes of ST. Unlike SB, ST does not occur without a reason. The cause of ST ranges from something as simple as anxiety to issues as complex as heart failure. Other possible causes of ST are anger, anemia, amphetamine use, caffeine consumption, cocaine use, exercise, fever, fright, hypotension, hypoxia, nicotine use, and pain.

Patients exhibiting ST are placed on a cardiac monitor and the underlying cause of the rhythm is treated.

SINUS ARRHYTHMIA

Sinus arrhythmia is similar to SR. It is also referred to as sinus dysrhythmia. All parameters are the same as SR except regularity. See Exhibit 6.4 and EKG 6.7 for details.

Regularity: R-R intervals have a slight variation that changes with the patient's respirations. The rhythm is slightly irregular.

Rate: Atrial and ventricular rates are equal. (The number of P waves is the same as the number of QRS complexes displayed on the EKG strip.)

Heart rate: 60–100 bpm, but may dip lower.

P wave: All P waves in the strip have a similar, uniform appearance. There is one P wave prior to each QRS complex.

PRI: 0.12–0.20 seconds, unchanging from beat to beat.

QRS: 0.04–0.10 seconds.

EXHIBIT 6.4 Characteristics of sinus arrhythmia.

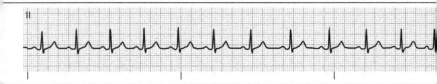

EKG 6.7 Sinus arrhythmia. This strip is longer than 6 seconds to depict the varying R-R intervals of this rhythm.

The most frequent causes of sinus arrhythmia are deep sleep and sleep apnea. Monitoring is generally all that is required regarding treatment.

═══════════════════════*FAST FACTS in a NUTSHELL*

- SR is normal, with a heart rate of 60 to 100.
- Other rhythms arise from the SA node, with varying rates.

7

The Atrial Rhythms

All cardiac cells hold the potential for automaticity, conductivity, and contractility. When cardiac cells located in the atrium outside of the conduction pathway get excited, conduct, and contract, abnormal beats and rhythms can occur.

In this chapter, you will learn:

1. The types of atrial rhythms
2. How to identify atrial rhythms on an EKG strip
3. The causes and treatments of atrial rhythms

Atrial rhythms are caused when cells in the atrium, located outside of the conduction pathway, get excited. The causes vary according to the specific rhythm. When a cell is excited, it has the ability to conduct an electrical current to the cells surrounding it. The neighboring cells pick up the signal and pass it on. Then, contractility among the excited cells can occur. (Keep in mind that electrical activity does not always mean mechanical activity.) When this circuit occurs outside of the normal atrial conduction pathway, abnormal beats, or rhythms, affecting the atria occur.

A PREMATURE ATRIAL CONTRACTION

A premature atrial contraction (PAC) occurs within an "underlying" rhythm, such as sinus rhythm (SR) with a PAC or sinus tachycardia (ST) with a PAC. It is one or two abnormal atrial beats that occur during a patient's regular rhythm. It is caused when an atrial cell outside of the conduction pathway gets excited and conducts an electrical stimulus that spreads to surrounding cells. The impulse is spread cell to cell until it reaches the AV node. It then follows the remaining normal conduction pathway through the Bundle of His, bundle branches, and Purkinje fibers. The result is an EKG tracing with an abnormal beat. See Figure 7.1 and EKG 7.1 for an illustration and an EKG strip example of a PAC.

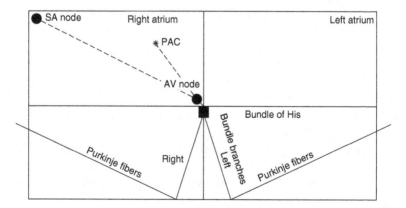

FIGURE 7.1   PAC.

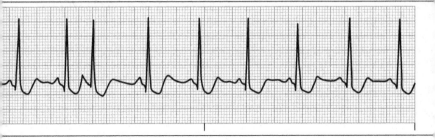

EKG 7.1 Sinus rhythm with a PAC.

The PAC will have a different P wave appearance from the underlying rhythm. The PRI is also often different. All parameters are dependent upon the underlying rhythm. See Exhibit 7.1 for detailed characteristics to identify a PAC.

Potential causes of PACs are alcohol intake, anxiety, atrial enlargement, congestive heart failure (CHF), digitalis toxicity, hypoxia, and stimulant use. If a cause can be determined, it is treated according to current medical guidelines.

Regularity: R-R intervals will vary dependent upon the position of the PAC within the strip. The rhythm is irregular.
Rate: Atrial and ventricular rates are equal, although not all P waves may be visualized.
Heart rate: Dependent on the underlying rhythm.
P wave: There is often one P wave prior to each QRS complex, depending on the underlying rhythm. The P wave of the PAC will look different than the P waves of the underlying rhythm. The P wave of the PAC may be flattened, notched, or hidden in the T wave. If visualized, the P wave will be upright in lead II.
PRI: 0.12–0.20 seconds. The PRI of the PAC is often different from that of the underlying rhythm, if it is measurable.
QRS: 0.04–0.10 seconds. It is the same in the PAC as it is in the underlying rhythm because once the abnormal "beat" reaches the AV node, it follows the conduction pathway resulting in a similar QRS duration.

EXHIBIT 7.1 Characteristics of a PAC.

==========*FAST FACTS in a NUTSHELL*

- PACs are not life-threatening.
- A large portion of the general population has an occasional PAC:
  - They are usually asymptomatic.
  - They generally require no treatment.

WANDERING PACEMAKER

The term "wandering pacemaker" is an excellent description of what occurs in the atrium with this abnormal EKG rhythm. In a healthy heart with a normal conduction pathway, the SA node is the pacemaker of the heart. For patients in the rhythm of wandering pacemaker, there are two areas in the atrium competing as the pacemaker or "driver." One area may be the SA node, but not necessarily. Two other excited areas in the atrium may be involved. Either way, both spots want to "drive" the heart.

This results in a changing R-R interval. The P wave changes with the pacemaker site, as can the PRI. The QRS interval remains constant because once the impulse initiated by either pacemaker site reaches the AV node, it follows the remaining normal conduction pathway. Figure 7.2 depicts the competing pacemakers and their flow through the heart. Exhibit 7.2 explains the identifying characteristics of a "wandering pacemaker." EKG 7.2 is a strip identified as wandering pacemaker.

The main cause of a wandering pacemaker is a change in vagal tone. This can be caused by a recent myocardial infarction, congestive heart failure, coronary artery disease, or various other reasons. Digitalis toxicity is another cause. This rhythm may also be normal in a small population of patients.

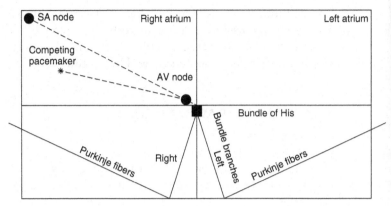

FIGURE 7.2 Illustration of conduction pathway of a wandering pacemaker rhythm.

Regularity: R-R intervals will have a slight variation. The rhythm is irregular.

Rate: Atrial and ventricular rates are equal. (The number of P waves is the same as the number of QRS complexes displayed on the EKG strip.)

Heart rate: Often 60–100 bpm; may be lower.

P wave: There is one P wave prior to each QRS complex. The P wave appearance will change with the pacemaker site initiating the beat.

PRI: 0.12–0.20 seconds. The PRI will vary with the pacemaker site initiating the beat.

QRS: 0.04–0.10 seconds. It is the same because once the "beat" reaches the AV node, it follows the conduction pathway resulting in a similar QRS duration.

EXHIBIT 7.2 Characteristics of a wandering pacemaker.

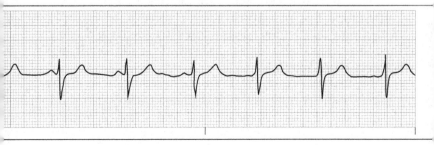

EKG 7.2 Wandering pacemaker.

This rhythm, while "abnormal," does not cause a major drop in cardiac output or cause many other symptoms. For this reason, it is not often treated and may even resolve on its own. If warranted, EKG monitoring will be continued.

PAROXYSMAL SUPRAVENTRICULAR TACHYCARDIA

Paroxysmal supraventricular tachycardia (PSVT) is when an area in the atrium gets superexcited. Chapter 2 discussed the electrical conduction in the heart and the conduction pathway. Also explained was that when a cardiac cell initiates impulses faster than the SA node, that area would take over as the "driver" of the heart.

This is what happens in PSVT. A superexcited area in the atrium initiates and conducts electrical impulses at a very fast rate of 150 to 250 per minute. The P waves are often lost or hidden in the flurry of activity and are not visualized on the EKG strip. The rhythm is regular, just extremely fast. The QRS is narrow due to the speed of the rhythm.

The great thing about EKG rhythms is that the names are often very descriptive of what is happening, electrically, in the heart. The P of PSVT is representative of paroxysmal, meaning "a sudden attack, a spasm, or a fit" (thefreedictionary .com/paroxysmal). This rhythm has a heart rate of 150 to 250 bpm, begins quickly, and is self-limiting. It might be captured on one 6-second strip or a few strips might be required. Either way, this rhythm bursts during an underlying rhythm and then stops (EKG 7.3). See Exhibit 7.3 for the identifying characteristics of PSVT.

Potential causes of PSVT are bronchodilators, caffeine intake, coronary artery disease, digitalis toxicity, rheumatic heart valve disease, stimulant use, and stress. A patient

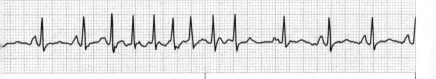

EKG 7.3   EKG sinus rhythm with a burst of PSVT.

Regularity: R-R intervals are constant during the burst of PSVT and may be constant within the underlying rhythm, depending on the underlying rhythm itself. However, the EKG strip will have a varying R-R interval due to the PSVT. The rhythm is overall irregular.

Rate: Atrial and ventricular rates may be equal, depending on the underlying rhythm. However, the P waves are rarely seen in the burst of PSVT. They are hidden, or "lost," due to the speed of the rhythm and the rapid depolarization of the ventricles. If visualized, the P waves will be upright in lead II.

Heart rate: Varies according to the underlying rhythm. It is 150–250 bpm in the burst of PSVT.

P wave: There is often one P wave prior to each QRS complex, depending on the underlying rhythm. The P waves are generally hidden during the burst of PSVT.

PRI: May be normal or abnormal, depending on the underlying rhythm. It will not often be measurable in the burst of PSVT due to the hidden P waves.

QRS: 0.04–0.10 seconds except during the burst of PSVT, which causes narrow QRS complexes due to the rapid depolarization of the ventricles.

EXHIBIT 7.3   Characteristics of a PSVT.

experiencing bursts of PSVT may complain of "heart racing," dizziness, near-syncope, and/or chest pain. Cardiac output can be affected during episodes of this fast heart rate, causing drops in blood pressure and perfusion.

Treatment depends on the underlying cause of the abnormal rhythm and may require extensive testing including electrophysiology (EP) studies.

SUPRAVENTRICULAR TACHYCARDIA

Supraventricular tachycardia (SVT) is simply PSVT without the P. It is sustained supraventricular tachycardia (EKG 7.4). It is not self-limiting and usually will not resolve without intervention. Exhibit 7.4 details the identifying characteristics of SVT.

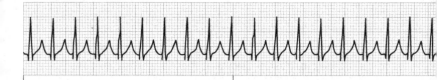

EKG 7.4   SVT.

Regularity: R-R intervals are constant. The rhythm is regular.
Rate: Atrial and ventricular rates are equal. However, the P waves are rarely seen because they are hidden, or "lost," due to the speed of the rhythm and the rapid depolarization of the ventricles. If seen, they will be upright in lead II.
Heart rate: 150–250 bpm.
P wave: Not often seen.
PRI: Not measurable due to the hidden P waves.
QRS: 0.04–0.10 seconds, usually narrow due to rapid ventricular depolarization.

EXHIBIT 7.4   Characteristics of SVT.

Possible causes of SVT are acute myocardial infarction, digitalis toxicity, dopamine or epinephrine administration, heart disease, hyperthyroidism, hypoxia, and mitral valve prolapse. Patients in SVT may complain of "heart racing," dizziness, near-syncope, nausea, and/or chest pain. Cardiac output is often severely reduced in SVT due to a drop in blood pressure and perfusion.

Treatment starts with simple vagal maneuvers in stable patients and progresses to adenosine administration. Unstable patients might be given adenosine but are more frequently quickly cardioverted to improve cardiac output. The underlying cause should be treated per medical guidelines. EP studies are often completed to provide valuable information on cardiac conduction.

MULTIFOCAL ATRIAL TACHYCARDIA

Multifocal atrial tachycardia (MAT) is an atrial rhythm that is often confused with the atrial rhythms of wandering pacemaker and atrial fibrillation. While the initial appearance of MAT on an EKG strip may seem similar to other rhythms (EKG 7.5), after reviewing Exhibit 7.5, its distinct identity will be revealed.

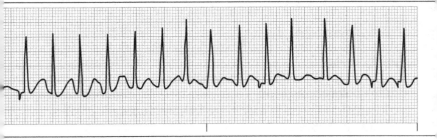

EKG 7.5   MAT.

Regularity: R-R intervals are not constant. The rhythm is irregular.
Rate: Atrial and ventricular rates are equal, but not all P waves may be visible.
Heart rate: Greater than 100.
P wave: There will be at least three different configurations because there are at least three different atrial pacemakers competing in this rhythm. The P waves may be notched or flattened and some may be hidden. If visualized, the P waves will be upright in lead II.
PRI: Changes with each pacemaker site.
QRS: 0.04–0.10 seconds.

EXHIBIT 7.5   Characteristics of MAT.

MAT is a rhythm that is not often encountered. It is a result of underlying medical conditions and will often resolve once the problem is treated. Conditions that can cause MAT are chronic lung disease, heart failure, methylxanthine toxicity, sepsis, and severe metabolic disturbances. Treatment revolves around the underlying cause.

ATRIAL FLUTTER

Atrial flutter (A flutter) is one of the easiest EKG rhythms to identify. Atrial activity is depicted in waves with a distinct saw-tooth appearance, known as "flutter waves," that replace P waves. In this cardiac rhythm, one excited area in the atrium sends out impulses at a rate of 240 to 350 per minute. The conductions spread through the atria to the AV node, which, acting as the "gatekeeper," lets only a certain amount of impulses through to continue down the conduction pathway. This action produces the "flutter waves" that are seen on the EKG strip.

Once the impulses pass thorough the AV node, they continue down through the ventricles normally resulting in a QRS that is of average width. See Exhibit 7.6 for the characteristics of A flutter.

Regularity: R-R intervals may be constant or irregular due to the number of atrial impulses conducted. The rhythm can be regular or irregular because the atrial rate is regular but the number of impulses allowed to pass through the AV node varies.
Rate: Atrial rate of 240–350 bpm. The ventricular rate is dependent upon the number of impulses that are conducted from the AV node.
Heart rate: Varies according to the number of atrial impulses conducted through the AV node.
P wave: None. Atrial activity is depicted as "flutter" waves, having a saw-tooth appearance.
PRI: None because there are no true P waves.
QRS: 0.04–0.10 seconds.

EXHIBIT 7.6 Characteristics of A flutter.

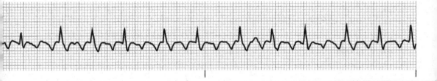

EKG 7.6 A flutter (3:1 and 2:1 conduction).

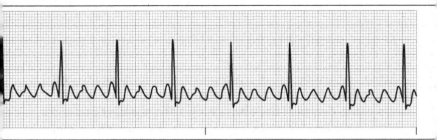

EKG 7.7 A flutter (4:1 conduction).

==*FAST FACTS in a NUTSHELL*

- Various conduction patterns may be seen in A flutter.
- Conduction rates can vary, with regularity, in a given EKG strip exhibiting A flutter.
  - For example, a strip may contain 3:1 and 2:1 conductions (see EKG 7.6).
  - A strip may also contain a straight 4:1 conduction (see EKG 7.7).
- An EKG rhythm strip should be identified as A flutter and if comfortable, conduction ratio can be noted but is not required.

A flutter can be caused by chronic cardiac ischemia, COPD, hypoxia, hypertension, pulmonary embolus, rheumatic heart disease, valve disease, and various other conditions. Treatment involves treating the underlying cause and controlling the ventricular rate. This is completed using antiarrhythmic drugs, such as flecainide, in conjunction with beta blockers or calcium channel blockers. Ablations via cardiac catheters are also frequently performed by electrophysiologists to manage A flutter.

ATRIAL FIBRILLATION

Atrial fibrillation (A fib) is another rhythm that involves multiple excited atrial cells. In this rhythm, the cells are spreading electrical impulses all over the chamber and the atria never depolarize as a whole. It is electrical chaos and the atria do not fully contract in a synchronized fashion. One visualization technique for A fib is a quivering Jell-O mold.

This action, or lack thereof, causes lots of problems. The blood in the atria begins to swirl and, pooling in some areas, has the potential for clot formation. Atrial kick is lost because the atria do not contract as a whole, thus lowering cardiac output by as much as 25%. Exhibit 7.7 describes the EKG strip characteristics of A fib.

========================FAST FACTS in a NUTSHELL

- A fib lacks P waves.
- The fibrillation line can be described as either fine (EKG 7.8) or coarse (EKG 7.9), but this is not required to identify the EKG strip as A fib.
- A fib is a stand-alone rhythm identification.

> *Regularity:* R-R intervals are not constant. The rhythm is irregular.
> *Rate:* Atrial rate is unmeasurable. The ventricular rate varies with the number of impulses conducted.
> *Heart rate:* Less than 100 bpm is referred to as controlled, more than 100 bpm is uncontrolled.
> *P wave:* None; chaotic fibrillation waves are seen.
> *PRI:* None; there are no P waves.
> *QRS:* 0.04–0.10 seconds.

EXHIBIT 7.7 Characteristics of A fib.

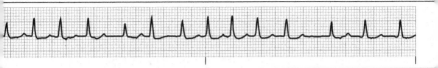

EKG 7.8 A fib with a fine fibrillation line.

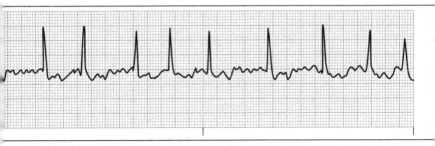

EKG 7.9 A fib with a coarse fibrillation line.

A fib may be caused by acute myocardial infarction, COPD, digitalis toxicity, hypoxia, hypertension, rheumatic valve disease, stimulant use, and thyrotoxicosis, along with various other conditions.

Treatment involves managing the underlying cause and controlling the ventricular rate. This is completed using beta blockers and/or calcium channel blockers. Digoxin (provided the patient is not dig-toxic), flecainide, and amiodarone may also be considered for the management of A fib. Cardioversion is a standard treatment, occurring on either an inpatient or outpatient basis. An ablation via a cardiac catheter may also be performed by an electrophysiologist.

FAST FACTS in a NUTSHELL

- Anticoagulation is critical in patients experiencing A fib due to the acute risk of thrombus formation in the atria.
  - Heparin, intravenous and subcutaneous, can be used.
  - Warfarin (Coumadin) is also frequently prescribed.
- Dabigatran (Pradaxa) and rivaroxaban (Xarelto) can both be used to anticoagulate patients.

8

The Junctional Rhythms

Junctional rhythms originate from the AV node or its immediate surrounding area. They occur because the SA node has failed or because the impulse coming from the nodal area is faster than that of the SA node.

In this chapter, you will learn:

1. The types of junctional rhythms
2. How to identify a junctional rhythm on an EKG strip
3. Possible causes and treatments of junctional rhythms

Junctional rhythms have distinct characteristics, most concerning the P wave. Impulses originate in the AV node and surrounding cells, thus changing the appearance of the P wave seen on an EKG strip. The P wave of a heartbeat originating in the "junction" will be inverted (upside down) in lead II and appear directly before or immediately after the QRS. The P wave may also be absent. The latter occurs when the atria depolarize at the same time as the QRS and the electrical activity within the atria is "overshadowed" by the electrical activity of the ventricles.

The appearance, or lack, of a P wave with a junctional beat is due to the retrograde conduction of the electrical impulse. It starts in the AV node area and then follows the normal electrical conduction pathway down through the Bundle of His, the bundle branches, and the Purkinje fibers. While this is going on, the impulse is also spreading up to the atria. See Figure 8.1 for a detailed anatomic drawing of retrograde conduction.

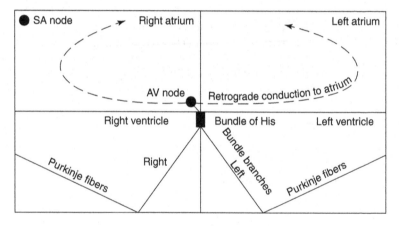

FIGURE 8.1 Anatomic drawing of retrograde conduction.

PREMATURE JUNCTIONAL CONTRACTION (PJC)

A PJC is similar to a premature atrial contraction (PAC). It is a premature contraction that occurs before the next expected regular beat; however, a PJC originates from an excited area in or near the AV node (EKG 8.1). Exhibit 8.1 describes the characteristics of a PJC.

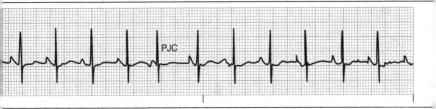

EKG 8.1 ST with a PJC.

> *Regularity:* R-R intervals will vary dependent upon the position of the PJC within the strip. The rhythm is **irregular**.
> *Rate:* Atrial and ventricular rates are equal, although not all P waves may be visualized.
> *Heart rate:* Dependent on the underlying rhythm.
> *P wave:* The P wave may be absent. If visualized, the P wave will be inverted in lead II and could come before or after the QRS.
> *PRI:* If the inverted P wave comes before the QRS, the PRI will be < 0.12 seconds.
> *QRS:* 0.04–0.10 seconds. It is the same in the PJC as it is in the underlying rhythm because once the abnormal "beat" reaches the AV node, and/or Bundle of His, it follows the normal conduction pathway resulting in a similar QRS duration.

EXHIBIT 8.1 Characteristics of a PJC.

Possible causes of PJCs are acute myocardial infarction, cardiac ischemia, congestive heart failure, digitalis toxicity, hypoxia, and stimulant use. Treatment is based on the underlying cause. PJCs themselves are not life-threatening.

JUNCTIONAL RHYTHM

Junctional rhythm originates from the AV node or its immediate surrounding area (Figure 8.2 and Exhibit 8.2) and EKG 8.2. It most often occurs when the SA node has failed as the "pacemaker" of the heart.

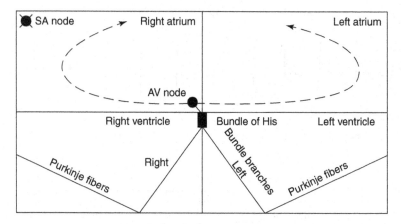

FIGURE 8.2 The heart with a junctional rhythm conduction pathway.

Regularity: This rhythm is **regular**.
Rate: Atrial and ventricular rates are equal, although the P waves may not be visualized.
Heart rate: 40–60 bpm.
P wave: The P wave may be absent. If visualized, the P wave will be inverted in lead II and could come before or after the QRS.
PRI: If the inverted P wave comes before the QRS, the PRI will be < 0.12.
QRS: 0.04–0.10 seconds.

EXHIBIT 8.2 Characteristics of junctional rhythm.

Possible causes of a junctional rhythm are acute myocardial infarction, beta blocker use, digitalis toxicity, increased vagal tone, and scarring around the SA node. Treatment may be based on the underlying cause but might not be required. Some patients tolerate a junctional rhythm well. Atropine can be given to increase the rate. Positive inotropes and pacemakers may also be utilized if the patient becomes symptomatic.

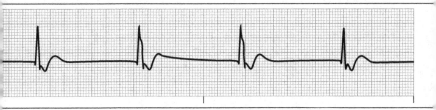

EKG 8.2 Junctional rhythm.

ACCELERATED JUNCTIONAL RHYTHM

An accelerated junctional rhythm occurs when the AV node and/or its immediate surrounding cells initiate an electrical impulse faster than that of the SA node. Conduction occurs in the same retrograde fashion as junctional rhythm. Exhibit 8.3 explains the characteristics of an accelerated junctional rhythm.

Regularity: This rhythm is **regular.**
Rate: Atrial and ventricular rates are equal, although the P waves may not be visualized.
Heart rate: 60–100 bpm.
P wave: The P wave may be absent. If visualized, the P wave will be inverted in lead II and could come before or after the QRS.
PRI: If the inverted P wave comes before the QRS, the PRI will be < 0.12.
QRS: 0.04–0.10 seconds.

EXHIBIT 8.3 Characteristics of an accelerated junctional rhythm.

Possible causes of an accelerated junctional rhythm are acute myocardial infarction, digitalis toxicity, isoproterenol (Isuprel) infusion, postoperative cardiac valve replacement, and/or increased vagal tone. Treatment would be based on the underlying cause but might not be required.

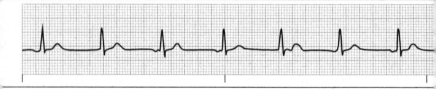

EKG 8.3   Accelerated junctional rhythm.

JUNCTIONAL TACHYCARDIA

Junctional tachycardia occurs when the AV node and/or its immediate surrounding cells initiate an electrical impulse faster than that of the SA node. It is similar to an accelerated junctional rhythm (EKG 8.3) with the exception of rate. Conduction occurs in the same retrograde fashion. Exhibit 8.4 explains the characteristics of junctional tachycardia.

Regularity: This rhythm is **regular.**
Rate: Atrial and ventricular rates are equal, although the P waves may not be visualized.
Heart rate: 100–180 bpm.
P wave: The P wave may be absent. If visualized, the P wave will be inverted in lead II and could come before or after the QRS.
PRI: If the inverted P wave comes before the QRS, the PRI will be < 0.12.
QRS: 0.04–0.10 seconds.

EXHIBIT 8.4   Characteristics of junctional tachycardia.

Possible causes of junctional tachycardia are acute myocardial infarction, digitalis toxicity, isoproterenol (Isuprel) infusion, and postoperative cardiac valve replacement. Treatment would be based on the underlying cause. Beta-adrenergic blockers and calcium channel blockers are often used to control the rate of junctional tachycardia (EKG 8.4).

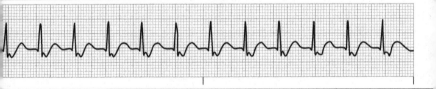

EKG 8.4 Junctional tachycardia.

═══════════════════════*FAST FACTS in a NUTSHELL*

- Junctional rhythm, accelerated junctional rhythm, and junctional tachycardia are very similar rhythms.
- The main difference among the three is the heart rate.

9

The Ventricular Rhythms

Ventricular rhythms originate from the ventricles. They occur either because the SA node and AV node have failed or because an area located within the ventricles gets excited and initiates impulses faster than the SA node.

In this chapter, you will learn:

1. The types of ventricular rhythms
2. How to identify a ventricular rhythm on an EKG strip
3. The causes and treatments of ventricular rhythms

Ventricular rhythms have distinct characteristics. Unlike the junctional rhythms, the QRS is different. The QRS of a beat that originates in the ventricle is wide and bizarre. It measures greater than 0.12 seconds in time. These impulses spread cell to cell, not via the electrical conduction pathway, therefore taking longer to complete a cycle. See Figure 9.1 for a diagram depicting an impulse originated in the ventricle.

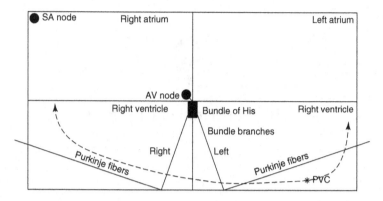

FIGURE 9.1   An electrical impulse originating in the ventricle.

The P wave is not seen on an EKG strip when the beat is ventricular in origin because the atria should be depolarizing at the same time as the ventricles. It is not known for sure if the atria actually depolarize when an impulse is generated from the ventricle. It may vary with each patient. Perfusion is not often associated with premature ventricular contractions (PVCs). For these reasons, PVCs are not generally counted when calculating the rate of a rhythm strip.

PREMATURE VENTRICULAR CONTRACTIONS

A PVC is a single impulse that is generated by the ventricle. It occurs before the next expected beat of the underlying rhythm. It is evidenced on the EKG strip by a wide, bizarre QRS. No P wave is seen during this beat. The rhythm is identified by stating the underlying rhythm and the PVC. See EKGs 9.1 and 9.2 for examples of EKG strips depicting a PVC. Exhibit 9.1 lists the characteristics of a PVC.

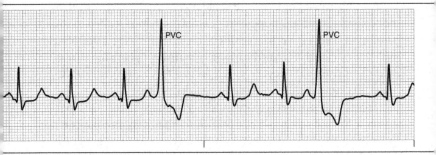

EKG 9.1 Sinus rhythm with two PVCs.

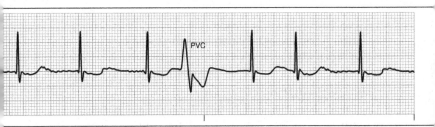

EKG 9.2 A fib with a PVC.

Regularity: R-R intervals will vary dependent upon the position of the PVC within the strip. The rhythm is **irregular.**
Rate: Dependent on the underlying rhythm.
Heart rate: Dependent on the underlying rhythm. PVCs are not counted when calculating the heart rate.
P wave: None seen in the impulse related to the PVC. The measurement of the remaining P waves will be dependent upon the underlying rhythm.
PRI: None seen in the impulse related to the PVC.
QRS: The QRS of the PVC will be > 0.12 seconds and wide and bizarre. The measurement of the remaining QRS complexes will be dependent on the underlying rhythm and is often normal.

EXHIBIT 9.1 Characteristics of a PVC.

Possible causes of PVCs are acute myocardial infarction, alcohol consumption, aminophylline, cardiac ischemia, caffeine consumption, congestive heart failure, digitalis toxicity, electrolyte imbalances, hypoxia, medications containing ephedrine, stress, stimulant use, and tricyclic antidepressants. Occasionally, PVCs have no cause at all, occurring in healthy people.

Treatment is based on the underlying cause. Tests are performed to rule out medical conditions that may predispose a patient to PVCs. However, PVCs themselves are not generally considered life-threatening.

═══════════════════════════*FAST FACTS in a NUTSHELL*

- PVCs can occur as a single impulse, or "beat," originating from one exited area known as a "focus."
- PVCs can also occur in various patterns and groups.
- If more than one PVC is observed in an EKG strip, they may originate from more than one focus.
- If more than one area is initiating PVCs, the ectopic (early) complexes will have different appearances on the EKG strip in relation to the focus that was the origination point.
- See EKGs 9.3 through 9.8 for EKG strips depicting examples of such PVCs.

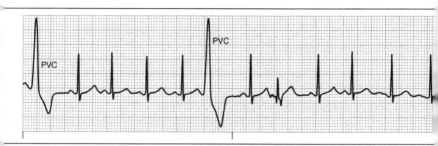

EKG 9.3   Sinus rhythm with unifocal PVCs.

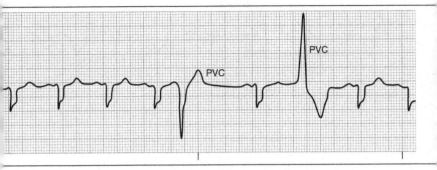

EKG 9.4 Sinus rhythm with a wide QRS (0.12 seconds) and multifocal PVCs.

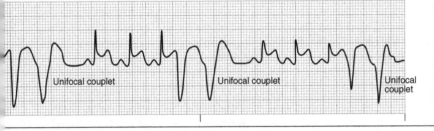

EKG 9.5 Sinus rhythm with an elevated ST segment and unifocal couplets.

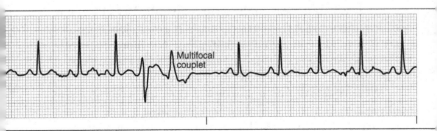

EKG 9.6 Sinus rhythm with a multifocal couplet.

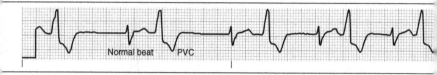

EKG 9.7 Bigeminal PVCs (bigeminy).

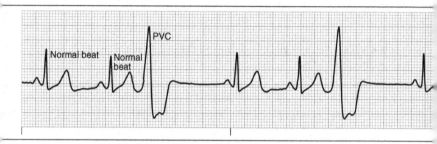

EKG 9.8 Trigeminal PVCs (trigeminy).

PVCs are identified as either unifocal (originating from one ventricular focus) or multifocal (originating from more than one ventricular focus). If PVCs occur in pairs, they are referred to as a couplet.

Couplets can be unifocal or multifocal. If every other beat on an EKG strip is identified as a PVC, it is termed bigeminy. When every third beat on the strip is identified as a PVC, it is called trigeminy. A rhythm strip depicting every fourth beat as a PVC would be known as quadreminy. The more frequently PVCs occur, the more life-threatening the rhythm becomes. Couplets are more dangerous than single PVCs.

When PVCs occur in a series of three or more at a rate of greater than 100 bpm, they are considered a "run" of ventricular tachycardia. The longer the runs last, the more life-threatening the abnormality.

VENTRICULAR TACHYCARDIA

Ventricular tachycardia (V-tach or VT) occurs when an excited area of the ventricle initiates electrical impulses at a very fast rate. The rhythm is life-threatening, as perfusion is very limited and may not be occurring at all. The ventricles are contracting so quickly that filling time is almost nonexistent. A series of three or more, wide, bizarre QRS complexes is noted on the EKG strip. The longer a run lasts, the more dangerous it becomes. See Exhibit 9.2 for the characteristics of VT. See EKGs 9.9 to 9.11 for examples.

Regularity: R-R intervals are constant. The rhythm is **regular**. If a run of VT occurs in a strip containing an underlying rhythm, the entire strip will be irregular but the VT will be regular and countable. The regularity of the underlying rhythm depends on the identification of the rhythm.
Rate: Atrial rate is unmeasurable. Ventricular rate > 100 bpm, generally 150–260 bpm. If a run of VT occurs in a strip containing an underlying rhythm, the rate will be dependent on the underlying rhythm.
Heart rate: > 100 bpm. If a run of VT occurs in a strip containing an underlying rhythm, the rate will be dependent upon the underlying rhythm.
P wave: None. If a run of VT occurs in a strip containing an underlying rhythm, the measurement of the remaining P waves will be dependent upon the underlying rhythm.
PRI: None. If a run of VT occurs in a strip containing an underlying rhythm, the measurement of the remaining PRIs will be dependent upon the underlying rhythm.
QRS: > 0.12 seconds; wide and bizarre. If a run of VT occurs in a strip containing an underlying rhythm, the measurement of the remaining QRS complexes will be dependent on the underlying rhythm.

EXHIBIT 9.2 Characteristics of VT.

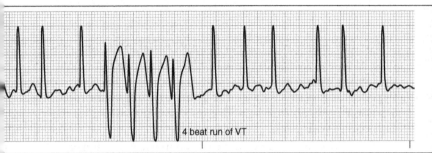

4 beat run of VT

EKG 9.9 A-fib with a four-beat run of VT.

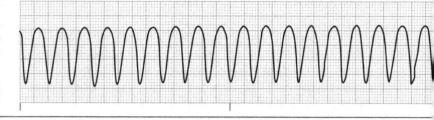

EKG 9.10   VT.

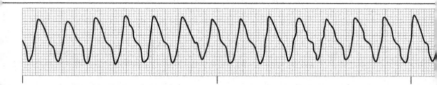

EKG 9.11   VT.

═══════════════*FAST FACTS in a NUTSHELL*

- VT can be life-threatening.
- If this rhythm is identified, immediately assess the patient.

Possible causes of VT are acute myocardial infarction, cardiac ischemia, congestive heart failure, cocaine or methamphetamine overdose, digitalis toxicity, electrolyte imbalances, hypoxia, and valve disease. The patient requires immediate attention to determine hemodynamic stability, which is the first step in treatment.

If the patient is stable, tests are completed to determine the cause of the VT. Correctable causes are treated and the patient is constantly monitored. Amiodarone or lidocaine may be administered via IV infusion. Antiarrhythmic medications, such as amiodarone, dofetilide, flecainide, ibutilide, mexiletine, procainamide, and sotalol, can also be prescribed in attempts to control chronic stable VT. Cardioversion is frequently performed and catheter ablations are often considered for patients refractory to other interventions. Internal cardiac defibrillators are often implanted.

When patients exhibiting VT are hemodynamically unstable, immediate cardioversion is the most frequent action taken. For pulseless VT, advanced cardiovascular life support (ACLS) guidelines should be followed. This begins with the initiation of CPR and immediate defibrillation. Refer to the American Heart Association's website (www.heart.org/HEARTORG/CPRAndECC/HealthcareProviders/Advanced CardiovascularLifeSupportACLS/AdvancedCardiovascular-Life-Support-ACLS_UCM_001280_SubHomePage.jsp) for details regarding complete ACLS guidelines.

VENTRICULAR FIBRILLATION

Ventricular fibrillation (V-fib or VF) is life-threatening. In fact, the patient is essentially dead. No perfusion is occurring with this rhythm and the heart is not "beating." During VF, several excited areas in the ventricles are initiating impulses at the same time. The electrical impulses are spread to localized cells and the ventricles are never depolarized as a whole. No conduction to the atria or mechanical contraction of the heart occurs. The heart is "fibrillating" or "jiggling." Imagine a tall Jell-O mold "jiggling" on a plate on top of a table someone has just bumped. This is what the heart does during VF. See Figure 9.2 for a diagram depicting a heart in VF, Exhibit 9.3 for the characteristics of VF on an EKG strip, and EKGs 9.12 and 9.13.

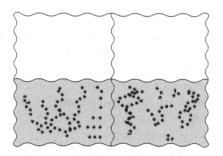

FIGURE 9.2 Diagram of a heart in VF (quivering).

Regularity: No measurable R-R interval. This rhythm is **irregular**.
Rate: Atrial and ventricular rates are unmeasurable.
Heart rate: Cannot be calculated.
P wave: None.
PRI: None.
QRS: No true QRS. Only fibrillation waves are seen.

EXHIBIT 9.3 Characteristics of VF.

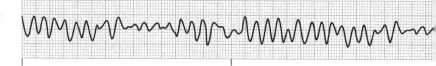

EKG 9.12 VF.

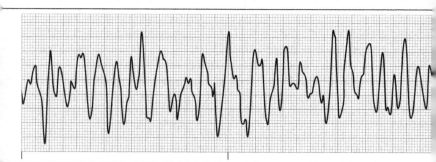

EKG 9.13 VF.

=====================================*FAST FACTS in a NUTSHELL*

- VF is fatal.
- If this rhythm is identified, immediately assess the patient, initiate CPR, and provide immediate defibrillation.

Possible causes of VF are acute myocardial infarction or ischemia, aortic dissection, cardiomyopathy, drowning, electrocution, electrolyte imbalances, hypoxia, pericardial tamponade, pulmonary embolism, R-on-T phenomenon, tension pneumothorax, and valve disease.

The treatment of VF follows ACLS guidelines beginning with the initiation of CPR and immediate defibrillation and progressing to the treatment of the cause. VF is often fatal. Refer to the American Heart Association's website (www.heart .org/HEARTORG/CPRAndECC/HealthcareProviders/ AdvancedCardiovascularLifeSupportACLS/Advanced Cardiovascular-Life-Support-ACLS_UCM_001280_SubHome Page.jsp) for details regarding complete ACLS guidelines.

IDIOVENTRICULAR RHYTHM

An idioventricular rhythm occurs when the SA node and AV node have failed. The ventricles take over as the "pacemaker" of the heart. The rate is slow. This is generally not considered a stable rhythm because the ventricular cells often quickly fail as impulse generators and there is a great potential for complete cardiac failure. Perfusion is not adequate related to the rate. See Exhibit 9.4 for the characteristics of an idioventricular rhythm and EKG 9.14.

Possible causes of an idioventricular rhythm are acidosis, acute myocardial infarction, emergence from cardiac arrest, and hypoxia.

> *Regularity:* This rhythm is **regular**.
> *Rate:* No atrial rate is noted. R-R intervals are generally regular.
> *Heart rate:* 20–40 bpm, could become slower with cardiac demise.
> *P wave:* None.
> *PRI:* None.
> *QRS:* Wide and bizarre; > 0.12 seconds.

EXHIBIT 9.4   Characteristics of an idioventricular rhythm.

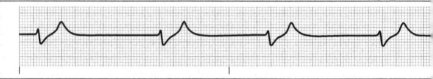

EKG 9.14   Idioventricular rhythm.

Treatment of an idioventricular rhythm includes IV medications such as epinephrine, dopamine, and/or isoproterenol. Ventricular pacing may be required. Beta blockers and calcium blockers should not be given to patients exhibiting an idioventricular rhythm because they could further slow the heart rate.

ACCELERATED IDIOVENTRICULAR RHYTHM

Accelerated idioventricular rhythm occurs when an area in the ventricles is initiating electrical impulses faster than that of the SA node. Patients are often asymptomatic requiring minimal intervention. See Exhibit 9.5 for the characteristics of an accelerated idioventricular rhythm and EKG 9.15.

> *Regularity:* This rhythm is **regular**.
> *Rate:* No atrial rate is noted. R-R intervals are generally regular.
> *Heart rate:* 40–100 bpm.
> *P wave:* None, as the atria (if functioning electrically) are depolarizing at a similar time as the ventricles.
> *PRI:* None, as no P waves are visible.
> *QRS:* Wide and bizarre; > 0.12 seconds.

EXHIBIT 9.5   Characteristics of an accelerated idioventricular rhythm.

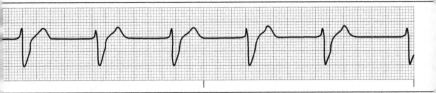

EKG 9.15 Accelerated idioventricular rhythm.

The possible causes of an accelerated idioventricular rhythm are cocaine overdose, digitalis toxicity, dilated cardiomyopathy, electrolyte imbalances, myocardial ischemia, and spinal anesthesia. Treatment of this rhythm revolves around treatment of the underlying cause. It may even resolve on its own, particularly in the case of myocardial ischemia reperfusion. Atropine might be considered if the patient becomes symptomatic.

10

Heart Block

Heart block is related to a problem in the AV node and/or its surrounding area. The causes of heart block vary but all result in a communication delay between the atria and the ventricles. When there is no electrical activity in the heart, it is termed asystole.

In this chapter, you will learn:

1. The types of heart block
2. How to identify heart block on an EKG strip
3. The causes and treatments of heart block
4. How to identify asystole
5. The causes and treatments of asystole

There are several types of heart block. Each has its own distinct characteristics. However, every rhythm that involves a heart block is caused by a problem with the AV node or its immediate surrounding cardiac cells. (Note: When AV node is stated, the area immediately around the AV node is included.) Communication between the atria and ventricles is disrupted because there is a breakdown in the normal electrical conduction pathway. The resulting abnormalities are observed on the EKG strip as prolonged PR intervals, changes in the P wave to QRS ratio, and, in some instances, QRS duration. The P waves remain upright in lead II and are similar in appearance with heart blocks because the SA node is initiating the impulses to the AV node normally even though the AV node is not functioning properly.

FIRST-DEGREE HEART BLOCK (I° HB)

1° HB occurs because there is a delay of the electrical impulse down the pathway as it encounters the AV node. The signal seems to get "hung up" and results in a lengthening of the PRI. The P wave to QRS ratio remains 1:1. Once the impulse leaves the AV node, it proceeds normally down the conduction pathway resulting in a QRS of normal duration. See Figure 10.1 for a diagram depicting the electrical pathway of a rhythm with a 1° HB. Exhibit 10.1 lists the characteristics of 1° HB and EKG 10.1 is an example of an EKG strip exhibiting this rhythm.

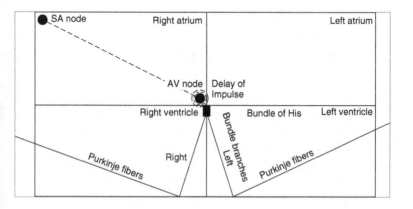

FIGURE 10.1 Electrical conduction pathway of 1° HB.

> *Regularity:* Depends on the underlying rhythm but R-R intervals are often consistent throughout the EKG strip. Most often the rhythm is **regular.**
> *Rate:* Atrial and ventricular rates are equal. (The number of P waves is the same as the number of QRS complexes displayed on the EKG strip.)
> *Heart rate:* Dependent upon the underlying rhythm.
> *P wave:* P waves have a similar, uniform appearance. There is one P wave prior to each QRS complex.
> *PRI:* > 0.20 seconds, unchanging from beat to beat.
> *QRS:* 0.04–0.10 seconds.

EXHIBIT 10.1   Characteristics of 1° HB.

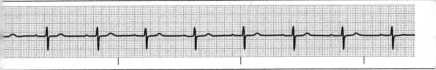

EKG 10.1   Sinus rhythm with 1° HB.

Some possible causes of 1° HB are acute myocardial infarction, antiarrhythmic medications, changes in vagal tone, conduction system disease of the heart, coronary artery disease, digitalis toxicity, rheumatic fever, and various infectious diseases. This conduction delay is generally well tolerated by patients and rarely requires intervention. Continued monitoring is often all that is performed with this condition. Other care provided would be centered on the treatment of the underlying cause, if deemed medically necessary.

SECOND-DEGREE HEART BLOCK (2° HB)

═══════════════════════════*FAST FACTS in a NUTSHELL*

- There are two types of 2° HB:
  - Mobitz type I (Wenckebach)
  - Mobitz type II

- In both types, impulses are generated by the SA node, resulting in P waves. However, the AV node fails to conduct all of them, causing an occasional loss of signal to the ventricles.
- This loss of conduction results in more P waves than QRS complexes observed on the EKG strip.

2° HB, Mobitz Type I (Wenckebach)

This type of heart block has a repetitive pattern of P wave to QRS relationship. With 2° HB, Mobitz type I, there is a progressive lengthening of the PRI until finally a QRS is "dropped" or missing. This occurs because the time it takes for impulses initiated by the SA node to travel through the AV node progressively increases with each beat until the AV node stops transmitting. A signal is not conducted to the ventricles, so no QRS is seen for the beat in which the AV node stopped transmitting because the ventricles did not repolarize. After this loss of conduction, the pattern starts over again. See Exhibit 10.2 for the characteristics of 2° HB, Mobitz type I, and EKG 10.2 for an example of an EKG strip exhibiting this rhythm.

Regularity: This rhythm is **irregular.** However, a repetitive pattern is usually seen.
Rate: Atrial and ventricular rates are not equal. The atrial rate is faster than the ventricular rate related to the nonconducted impulses.
Heart rate: Generally, the ventricular rate will be < 60 bpm.
P wave: P waves have a similar, uniform appearance.
PRI: Gets progressively longer until a QRS is "dropped."
QRS: 0.04–0.10 seconds.

EXHIBIT 10.2   Characteristics of 2° HB, Mobitz type I (Wenckebach).

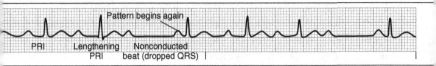

EKG 10.2   2° HB, Mobitz type I.

Possible causes of 2° HB, Mobitz type I are acute myocardial infarction, antiarrhythmic medications, cardiac surgery, changes in vagal tone, conduction system disease of the heart, digitalis toxicity, hyperkalemia, hypermagnesemia, rheumatic syndromes, and various infectious diseases. Treatment of 2° HB, Mobitz type I depends upon the patient. If asymptomatic, the treatments will center on uncovering the cause. If symptomatic, atropine may be given according to the American Heart Association (AHA) ACLS guidelines and could be coupled with external or internal pacing.

================================*FAST FACTS in a NUTSHELL*

- The QRS complexes of both types of 2° HB remain of normal duration.
- This occurs because the impulses that are conducted by the AV node to the ventricles follow the remaining normal conduction pathway.

2° HB, Mobitz Type II

This rhythm is extremely similar to 2° HB, Mobitz type I except it lacks the lengthening PRI. In 2° HB, Mobitz type II, the SA node initiates electrical impulses and sends them to the AV node via the conduction pathway. The AV node conducts some impulses to the ventricles but not all. This abnormality in the AV node results in more P waves than QRS complexes observed on the EKG strip. After the loss of conduction, the pattern starts over again. See Exhibit 10.3 for the characteristics of 2° HB, Mobitz type II, and EKG 10.3 for an example of an EKG strip exhibiting this rhythm.

Regularity: This rhythm is **irregular**. However, a repetitive pattern is usually seen.
Rate: Atrial and ventricular rates are not equal. The atrial rate is faster than the ventricular rate related to the nonconducted impulses.
Heart rate: Generally, the ventricular rate will be < 60 bpm.
P wave: P waves have a similar, uniform appearance.
PRI: Generally, 0.12–0.20 when measurable.
QRS: 0.04–0.10 seconds.

EXHIBIT 10.3   Characteristics of 2° HB, Mobitz type II.

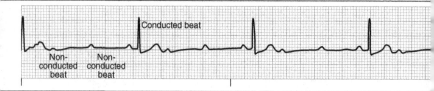

EKG 10.3   2° HB, Mobitz type II.

Possible causes of 2° HB, Mobitz type II are acute myocardial infarction, antiarrhythmic medications, cardiac surgery, conduction system disease of the heart, digitalis toxicity, hyperkalemia, hypermagnesemia, rheumatic syndromes, and various infectious diseases.

2° HB, Mobitz type II is more dangerous than 2° HB, Mobitz type I because it has the tendency to advance to 3° heart block (complete heart block). Pacing is initiated quickly and permanent pacemakers are almost always implanted in patients in 2° HB, Mobitz type II. Atropine may also be given but pacing is the gold standard of treatment.

3° HB

3° HB is also known as complete heart block. It is a very dangerous rhythm. There is a complete breakdown in the communication between the atria and the ventricles. The AV node is no longer conducting any of the impulses initiated by the SA node, causing the ventricles to initiate their own impulses. The result is no connection between the P waves and the QRS complexes. No PRI is measurable because none exists. The P waves are upright in lead II and similar in appearance, coming at regular intervals. The QRS complexes are > 0.12 seconds in duration because the ventricles are initiating their own impulses, which come at regular intervals. See Exhibit 10.4 for the characteristics of 3° HB, and EKG 10.4 for an example of an EKG strip exhibiting this rhythm.

Regularity: This rhythm is **regular.** P waves and QRS complexes occur at regular intervals, but not in relationship to one another.

Rate: Atrial and ventricular rates are not equal. The atrial rate is faster than the ventricular rate.

Heart rate: Generally, the ventricular rate will be < 40 bpm.

P wave: P waves have a similar, uniform appearance.

PRI: None because there is no relationship between the P waves and QRS complexes.

QRS: > 0.12 seconds.

EXHIBIT 10.4   Characteristics of 3° HB.

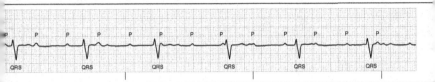

EKG 10.4   3° HB.

Possible causes of 3° HB are acute myocardial infarction, antiarrhythmic medications, cardiac surgery, conduction system disease of the heart, digitalis toxicity, hyperkalemia, hypoxia, rheumatic syndromes, and various infectious diseases.

3° HB is extremely dangerous. An important consideration is the cause of the block. Any possible interventions to resolve or counteract the cause should be performed. Pacing, frequently transvenous, is quickly initiated and permanent pacemakers are almost always implanted. Atropine may be given, but cautiously, as it may worsen certain cases of 3° HB. Isoproterenol may also be considered to increase the heart rate until pacing can be initiated.

ASYSTOLE

Asystole is the term used when there is no electrical activity in the heart. This heart is in complete failure and absolutely not moving. A straight line is seen on the rhythm strip (EKG 10.5). This patient is essentially dead and CPR must be initiated. AHA ACLS guidelines should be followed. The possible causes of asystole are varied; ranging from cardiac tamponade to acute myocardial infarction to acute trauma. Treatment attempts would center on uncovering and then resolving the cause.

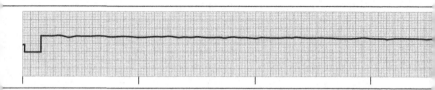

EKG 10.5 Asystole.

II

Pacing and Bundle Branch Blocks

When learning the basics of identifying EKG strips, it is important to focus on the most frequently seen rhythms and the most lethal. However, pacing and bundle branch blocks are two EKG strips that clinicians should be able to recognize.

In this chapter, you will learn:

1. How to identify a paced rhythm on an EKG strip
2. How to identify a bundle branch block on an EKG strip
3. The causes and treatments of bundle branch blocks

PACED RHYTHMS

As explained in previous chapters, there are several cardiac rhythms that require pacing as an intervention. The pacing may occur externally via pacing pads or internally via a temporary transvenous pacing catheter, epicardial pacing wires placed during cardiac surgery, or an implanted device such as a permanent pacemaker or an internal cardiac defibrillator (ICD).

════════════════════════*FAST FACTS in a NUTSHELL*

- No distinction is observed on the EKG strip regarding which pacing device or mode generates the electrical impulses.

Cardiac pacing can be performed in the atria and the ventricles. Both areas may require pacing; however, each area can be stimulated separately. The EKG strip will reflect which area is being electrically paced.

Pacing spikes are seen on the EKG strip prior to the corresponding complex of the chamber being paced. See EKG 11.1 for an example of ventricular pacing and EKG 11.2 for an example of AV pacing.

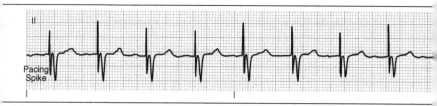

EKG 11.1 Ventricular pacing.

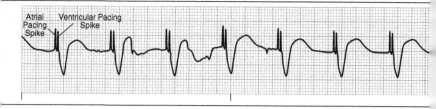

EKG 11.2 AV pacing.

When pacing spikes are observed on the EKG strip but not in the correct position in relationship to the rhythm complexes, the pacemaker needs to be adjusted. If a device fails to "capture," a pacing spike is seen but no P wave or QRS complex follows it. Generally, the output, or milliampere (mA), which is the electrical current the pacing device applies to the cardiac tissue, is increased until capture is noted on the EKG. Occasionally, if a temporary wire catheter is the device, it will be repositioned. See EKG 11.3 for an example of pacing that exhibits a failure to capture.

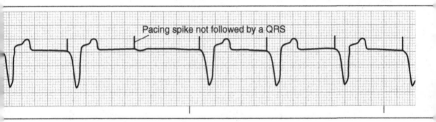

Pacing spike not followed by a QRS

EKG 11.3   Failure to capture.

When a device fails to "sense," a pacing spike is seen without correlation to a P wave or QRS complex. The pacing spike appears during a cardiac cycle, sometimes close to the T wave. The sensitivity of the pacing device is adjusted to correct this problem. Occasionally, a temporary pacing catheter will require repositioning to correct the problem. If no intervention with the settings or placement occurs, there is a high possibility that the R-on-T phenomenon will occur, which launches the patient into ventricular tachycardia (VT) or ventricular fibrillation (VF). Refer to EKG 11.4 for an example of pacing that exhibits failure to sense.

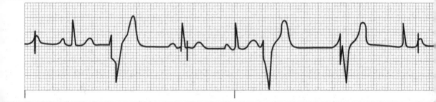

EKG 11.4 Failure to sense occurs where the pacing spikes are observed during intrinsic beats (1st, 4th, and 8th beats).

BUNDLE BRANCH BLOCK (BBB)

In a normal electrical conduction pathway, the bundle branches depolarize at the same time. When a BBB is present, either the left or right bundle branch depolarizes first. The electrical impulse takes longer to move through the other side. This causes a slight variation in the appearance of the QRS.

A BBB can occur on either side of the bundle branches. A right BBB (RBBB) is observed in EKG 11.5 and a left BBB (LBBB) in EKG 11.6. Both types of BBB can be difficult to observe in lead II.

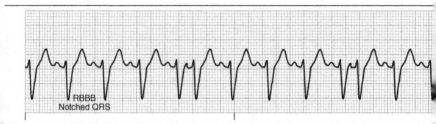

EKG 11.5 RBBB.

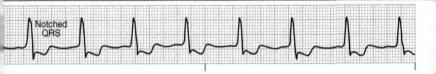

EKG 11.6 LBBB.

Some issues that cause BBB are acute myocardial infarction, cardiomyopathy, cardiac surgery, congestive heart failure, coronary artery disease, hypertension, pulmonary embolism, and valve disease. It can occur in healthy hearts, too. A BBB is not fatal, with some patients exhibiting no symptoms. A 12-lead EKG will be completed and cardiology will be consulted. Treatment may be deferred due to this reason but could involve pacemaker implantation and ventricular resynchronization if the patient becomes symptomatic.

Appendices

Appendix A: Practice Strips

Unless otherwise noted, consider all EKG strips 6 seconds.

Example:

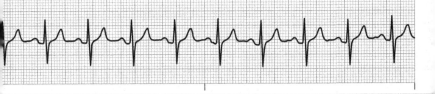

Regularity: <u>Yes</u>

Rate: <u>90</u>

P Waves: <u>Yes, 1 P wave for every QRS</u>

PRI: <u>0.16</u>

QRS: <u>0.08</u>

Identity: <u>SR</u>

1.

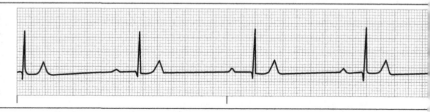

Regularity:_____

Rate:_____

P Waves:_____

PRI:_____

QRS:_____

Identity:_____

2.

Regularity:_____

Rate:_____

P Waves:_____

PRI:_____

QRS:_____

Identity:_____

3.

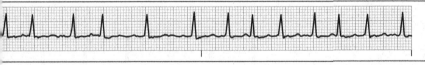

Regularity:_____

Rate:_____

P Waves:_____

PRI:_____

QRS:_____

Identity:_____

4.

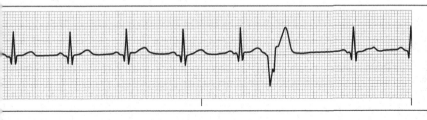

Regularity:_____

Rate:_____

P Waves:_____

PRI:_____

QRS:_____

Identity:_____

5.

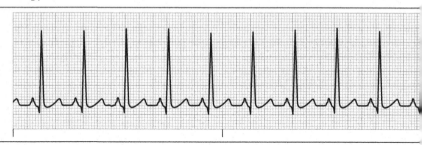

Regularity:_____

Rate:_____

P Waves:_____

PRI:_____

QRS:_____

Identity:_____

6.

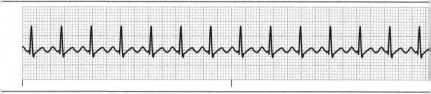

Regularity:_____

Rate:_____

P Waves:_____

PRI:_____

QRS:_____

Identity:_____

7.

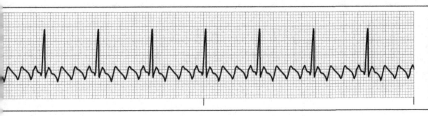

Regularity:_____

Rate:_____

P Waves:_____

PRI:_____

QRS:_____

Identity:_____

8.

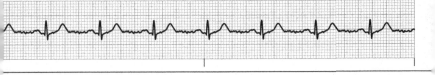

Regularity:_____

Rate:_____

P Waves:_____

PRI:_____

QRS:_____

Identity:_____

9.

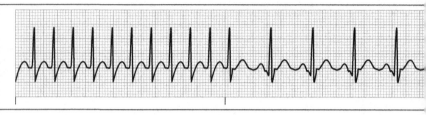

Regularity:_____

Rate:_____

P Waves:_____

PRI:_____

QRS:_____

Identity:_____

10.

Regularity:_____

Rate:_____

P Waves:_____

PRI:_____

QRS:_____

Identity:_____

11.

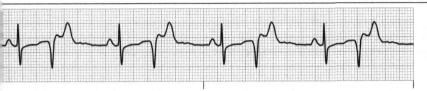

Regularity:_____

Rate:_____

P Waves:_____

PRI:_____

QRS:_____

Identity:_____

12.

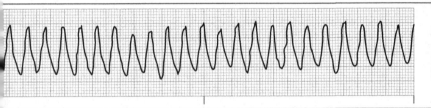

Regularity:_____

Rate:_____

P Waves:_____

PRI:_____

QRS:_____

Identity:_____

13.

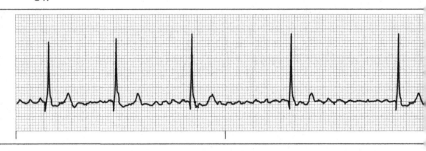

Regularity:_____

Rate:_____

P Waves:_____

PRI:_____

QRS:_____

Identity:_____

14.

Regularity:_____

Rate:_____

P Waves:_____

PRI:_____

QRS:_____

Identity:_____

15.

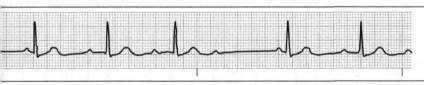

Regularity:_____

Rate:_____

P Waves:_____

PRI:_____

QRS:_____

Identity:_____

16.

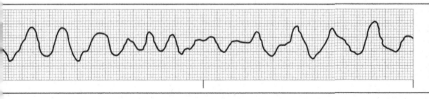

Regularity:_____

Rate:_____

P Waves:_____

PRI:_____

QRS:_____

Identity:_____

17.

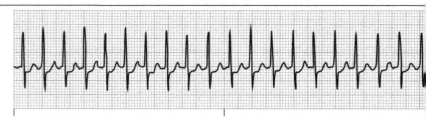

Regularity:_____

Rate:_____

P Waves:_____

PRI:_____

QRS:_____

Identity:_____

18.

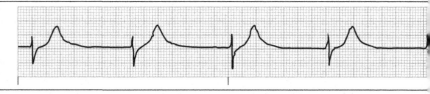

Regularity:_____

Rate:_____

P Waves:_____

PRI:_____

QRS:_____

Identity:_____

19.

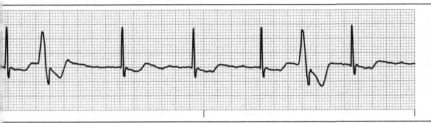

Regularity:_____

Rate:_____

P Waves:_____

PRI:_____

QRS:_____

Identity:_____

20.

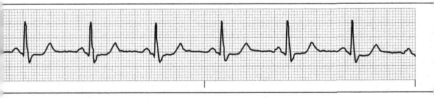

Regularity:_____

Rate:_____

P Waves:_____

PRI:_____

QRS:_____

Identity:_____

ANSWERS TO APPENDIX A

1. Regularity: <u>No</u>
Rate: <u>Cannot count</u>
P Waves: <u>None</u>
PRI: <u>N/A</u>
QRS: <u>Wide, irregular</u>
Identity: <u>VF</u>

2. Regularity: <u>Yes</u>
Rate: <u>40</u>
P Waves: <u>Yes, 1 P wave for each QRS</u>
PRI: <u>0.28</u>
QRS: <u>0.04</u>
Identity: <u>SB with 1° HB</u>

3. Regularity: <u>No</u>
Rate: <u>130</u>
P Waves: <u>No</u>
PRI: <u>N/A</u>
QRS: <u>0.06</u>
Identity: <u>A fib</u>

4. Regularity: <u>Underlying rhythm is regular, 1 ectopic beat</u>
Rate: <u>60</u>
P Waves: <u>Yes, 1 P wave for each QRS except for the ectopic beat</u>
PRI: <u>0.16</u>
QRS: <u>0.10, except the ectopic beat in which the QRS measures 0.40</u>
Identity: <u>SR with 1 PVC</u>

5. Regularity: <u>Yes</u>

Rate: <u>100</u>

P Waves: <u>Yes</u>

PRI: <u>0.12</u>

QRS: <u>0.08</u>

Identity: <u>SR</u>

6. Regularity: <u>Yes</u>

Rate: <u>140</u>

P Waves: <u>Yes, 1 P wave for every QRS</u>

PRI: <u>0.16</u>

QRS: <u>0.04</u>

Identity: <u>ST</u>

7. Regularity: <u>Yes</u>

Rate: <u>70</u>

P Waves: <u>No, flutter waves</u>

PRI: <u>N/A</u>

QRS: <u>0.04</u>

Identity: <u>A Flutter</u>

8. Regularity: <u>Yes</u>

Rate: <u>70</u>

P Waves: <u>Yes</u>

PRI: <u>0.16</u>

QRS: <u>0.04</u>

Identity: <u>SR</u>

9. Regularity: <u>Yes, in underlying rhythm. Yes in "burst."</u>

Rate: <u>Underlying rhythm rate is 80. "Burst" rate is approximately 200.</u>

P Waves: <u>Yes, 1 P wave for every QRS in the underlying rhythm. The P waves are "hidden" in the "burst."</u>

PRI: <u>0.16 in the underlying rhythm</u>

QRS: <u>0.04</u>

Identity: <u>SR with a burst of PSVT</u>

10. Regularity: <u>N/A</u>

Rate: <u>N/A</u>

P Waves: <u>N/A</u>

PRI: <u>N/A</u>

QRS: <u>N/A</u>

Identity: <u>Asystole</u>

11. Regularity: <u>Yes</u>

Rate: <u>40</u>

P Waves: <u>Yes, 1 P wave for every QRS in the underlying rhythm. No P waves noted in the abnormal beats.</u>

PRI: <u>0.16 in the underlying rhythm</u>

QRS: <u>0.08 in the underlying rhythm, 0.40 in the abnormal beats.</u>

Identity: <u>Bigeminal PVCs (Bigeminy)</u>

12. Regularity: <u>Yes</u>

Rate: <u>230</u>

P Waves: <u>No</u>

PRI: <u>N/A</u>

QRS: <u>0.20</u>

Identity: <u>VT</u>

13. Regularity: <u>Yes</u>

Rate: <u>40</u>

P Waves: <u>No</u>

PRI: <u>N/A</u>

QRS: <u>0.24</u>

Identity: <u>Idioventricular</u>

14. Regularity: <u>No</u>

Rate: <u>50</u>

P Waves: <u>No</u>

PRI: <u>N/A</u>

QRS: <u>0.08</u>

Identity: <u>A fib</u>

15. Regularity: <u>No</u>

Rate: <u>70 atrial, 50 ventricular</u>

P Waves: <u>Yes, occasionally more than 1 P wave for a QRS</u>

PRI: <u>Varies, progressively lengthening</u>

QRS: <u>0.04</u>

Identity: <u>2° HB, Mobitz type 1</u>

16. Regularity: <u>No</u>

Rate: <u>Unable to count</u>

P Waves: <u>No</u>

PRI: <u>N/A</u>

QRS: <u>Chaotic</u>
Identity: <u>VF</u>

17. Regularity: <u>Yes</u>
Rate: <u>200</u>
P Waves: <u>Hidden</u>
PRI: <u>N/A</u>
QRS: <u>0.04</u>
Identity: <u>SVT</u>

18. Regularity: <u>Yes</u>
Rate: <u>50</u>
P Waves: <u>No</u>
PRI: <u>N/A</u>
QRS: <u>0.08</u>
Identity: <u>Junctional</u>

19. Regularity: <u>No</u>
Rate: <u>50</u>
P Waves: <u>None</u>
PRI: <u>N/A</u>
QRS: <u>0.08 in underlying rhythm, wide and bizarre in abnormal beats</u>
Identity: <u>A fib with 2 PVCs</u>

20. Regularity: <u>Yes</u>
Rate: <u>60</u>
P Waves: <u>Yes, 1 P wave for every QRS</u>
PRI: <u>0.16</u>
QRS: <u>0.08</u>
Identity: <u>SR</u>

Appendix B: Practice Scenarios

Consider all EKG strips 6 seconds unless otherwise noted.

1. A patient presents to the clinic complaining of nausea and vomiting for 2 days. She is 38 years old and "feels terrible and tired." She has no medical history with the exception of a broken right arm as a child. She takes no medications and denies any recent use of over-the-counter medications. Her blood pressure is 89/58, heart rate is 45, and respirations are 16. You connect her to the monitor and this is the rhythm strip printed:

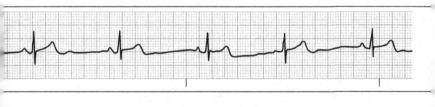

   What is the rhythm?_____

   What possible interventions may be utilized?_____

   _____

2. A 19-year-old male presents to the emergency department complaining of dizziness and nausea for the last 30 minutes.

He also states "My heart feels like it might jump out of my chest." His vital signs are blood pressure 98/60, heart rate 200, and respirations 22. When he is connected to the monitor, this is the patient's EKG strip:

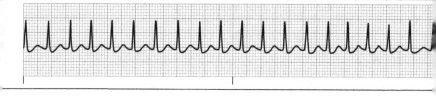

What is the rhythm?_____

What possible interventions may be utilized?_____

_____

3. You are working in a cardiology clinic. A 67-year-old man has come in for his first follow-up visit after permanent pacemaker implantation. He denies any problems. He is connected to the in-room monitor and this rhythm is observed:

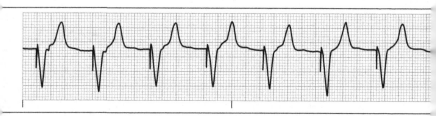

What is the rhythm?_____

What possible interventions may be utilized?_____

_____

4. A 99-year-old woman comes to the urgent care clinic after a day of feeling "not well." Her physical exam is negative and she denies any other symptoms. She has "never taken medications in my life." Her vital signs are within normal limits. Chest x-ray is clear. Upon connecting her to the EKG monitor, this rhythm is visualized:

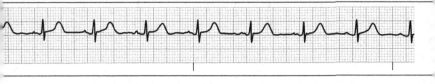

What is the rhythm?_____

What possible interventions may be utilized?_____

5. A patient is found down on the floor in her hospital room. She has no pulse and is not breathing. CPR is initiated. Once she is connected to the bi-phasic defibrillator/monitor, this rhythm is seen:

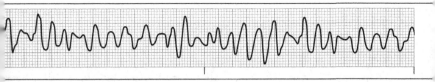

What is the rhythm?_____

What possible interventions may be utilized?_____

6. A 56-year-old male on your telemetry floor complains of shortness of breath. His vital signs are stable but his radial pulse feels "strange" when palpated. His EKG strips are reviewed and this rhythm is noted:

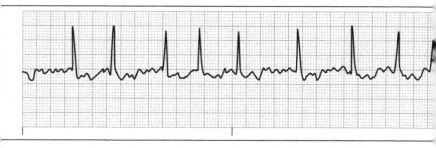

What is the rhythm?_____

What possible interventions may be utilized?_____

7. A 76-year-old woman in the heart catheterization lab recovery area status post one stent to the left anterior descending artery is complaining of her heart "skipping." An EKG strip is run:

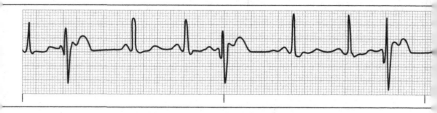

What is the rhythm?_____

What possible interventions may be utilized?_____

_____

8. A 19-year-old male presents to the clinic with a fever of 103°F. He complains of coughing, sneezing, and "gross" sputum for 2 days. His blood pressure is 110/71, heart rate 115, respirations 19. His EKG rhythm is evaluated:

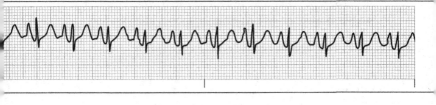

What is the rhythm?_____

What possible interventions may be utilized?_____

9. A 41-year-old man status post acute myocardial infarction is found down on the floor in the bathroom of his hospital room. He is unresponsive. No pulse is palpable and he is not breathing. CPR is initiated and he is immediately connected to a bi-phasic defibrillator/monitor. This is what is seen by the team:

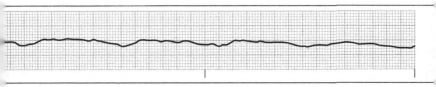

What is the rhythm?_____

What possible interventions may be utilized?_____

10. A 48-year-old woman is at the office for her annual check-up. She has been doing "okay" but does complain of "feeling a bit tired lately." She is not currently on any medications but does take a multivitamin and 500 mg of calcium each day. Her only medical history is a C-section 10 years ago that was uncomplicated. Her vital signs are stable. However, her rhythm strip reveals:

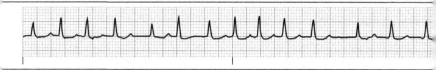

What is the rhythm?_____

What possible interventions may be utilized?_____

_____

ANSWERS TO APPENDIX B

1. This is SB. Uncovering the patient's prior baseline heart rate would be helpful. Possible interventions could be as simple as encouraging the patient to improve oral fluid intake and prescribing an antiemetic. An IV could be started and a bolus of IV fluid, such as normal saline or lactated Ringer's, might be given to improve patient symptoms, blood pressure, and heart rate. Follow-up in a few days should be recommended to monitor her symptoms and heart rate.

2. This is SVT. Possible interventions include attempting vagal maneuver, as long as the patient remains stable. However, since he might quickly become unstable, an IV should be inserted and preparations begun for the anticipated administration of adenosine. If he did become unstable, cardioversion is an option to utilize.

3. This patient is being ventricularly paced. No interventions would be needed if all other parameters of the device are functioning properly. The patient should continue his follow-up schedule.

4. This is SR. This patient has no remarkable conditions and should be referred to her primary physician for follow-up to today's visit and return back to the urgent care clinic for new or worsening complaints.

5. This is VF. The patient should be immediately defibrillated with 200 joules of electricity. CPR should be resumed immediately after the shock and advanced cardiovascular life support (ACLS) guidelines should be followed.

6. This is A fib. Cardiology should be consulted. Possible interventions to expect are rate control with medications such as beta blockers or calcium channel blockers, anticoagulation, and cardioversion.

7. This is SR with a PVC. She felt her heart "skip" because of the ventricular beat. Vital signs should be taken, a 12-lead EKG performed, and lab work drawn. A couple of isolated PVCs may not be lethal but could be precursors to a worsening cardiac condition.

8. This is ST. This young man's tachycardia is caused by his fever and infection/virus. Interventions to expect would be increasing oral fluids, chest x-ray, and possible antibiotics.

9. This is asystole. CPR must continue and ACLS guidelines must be followed.

10. This is A-fib. Cardiology should be consulted. Interventions to anticipate are anticoagulation along with beta blockers, calcium channel blockers, digoxin, flecainide, and/or amiodarone. Cardioversion is a standard treatment, occurring on either an inpatient or outpatient basis.

Bibliography

Ahrens, T. S., Prentice, D., & Kleinpell, R. M. (2010). *Critical care nursing certification: Preparation, review, and practice exams* (6th ed.). New York, NY: McGraw-Hill Medical.

Alspach, J. G. (2006). *Core curriculum for critical care nursing* (6th ed.). St. Louis, MO: Saunders Elsevier.

Beinhart, S. C. (2012, June). *Junctional rhythm*. Retrieved October 21, 2012, from www.emedicine.medscape.com/article/155146-overview

Budzikowski, A. S., Corsello, A. C., Daubert, J. P., Gaeta, T. J., Levine, M. D., & Shah, A. H. (2011, September). *Third-degree atrioventricular block*. Retrieved October 28, 2012, from www.emedicine.medscape.com/article/162007-overview#awaab6b2b3

Budzikowski, A. S., Corsello, A. C., Daubert, J. P., Gaeta, T. J., Levine, M. D., & Shah, A. H. (2011, September). *Third-degree atrioventricular block clinical presentation*. Retrieved October 28, 2012, from www.emedicine.medscape.com/article/162007-clinical

Budzikowski, A. S., Corsello, A. C., Daubert, J. P., Gaeta, T. J., Levine, M. D., & Shah, A. H. (2011, September). *Third-degree atrioventricular block treatment & management*. Retrieved October 28, 2012, from www.emedicine.medscape.com/article/162007-treatment

Bundle Branch Block. (2012, August). Retrieved October 29, 2012, from www.texasheartinstitute.org/HIC/Topics/Cond/bbblock.cfm?&RenderForPrint=1

Compton, S. J., Conrad, S. A., Setnik, G., deSouzza, I. S., & Ward, C. D. (2012, October). *Ventricular tachycardia.* Retrieved October 26, 2012, from www.emedicine.medscape.com/article/159075-overview

Compton, S. J., Conrad, S. A., Setnik, G., deSouzza, I. S., & Ward, C. D. (2012, October). *Ventricular tachycardia treatment & management.* Retrieved October 26, 2012, from www.emedicine.medscape.com/article/159075-treatment#aw2aab6b6b3

Dubin, D. (2000). *Rapid interpretation of EKG's* (6th ed.). Tampa, FL: Cover Publishing Company.

Fongoros, R. (2011, November). *Bundle branch block.* Retrieved October 29, 2012, from www.heartdisease.about.com/cs/arrhythmias/a/BBB.htm?p=1

Fongoros, R. (2011, November). *Bundle branch block - 2.* Retrieved October 29, 2012, from www.heartdisease.about.com/cs/arrhythmias/a/BBB_2.htm?p=1

Fongoros, R. (2011, November). *Bundle branch block - 3.* Retrieved October 29, 2012, from www.heartdisease.about.com/cs/arrhythmias/a/BBB_3.htm?p=1

Francis, J. (2009, September). *Idioventricular rhythms.* Retrieved October 26, 2012, from www.cardiophile.org/2009/09/idioventricular-rhythms/

Free Online Dictionary, Thesaurus, and Encyclopedia. Retrieved October 15, 2012, from www.thefreedictionary.com/Paroxysmal

Green, J. M., & Chiaramida, A. J. (2010). *12-Lead EKG confidence: A step-by-step guide* (2nd ed.). New York, NY: Springer Publishing Company.

Gross Cohn, E. (2009). *Flip and see ECG* (3rd ed.). St. Louis, MO: Mosby Jems Elsevier.

Hodgson, B. B., & Kizior, R. J. (2010). *Saunders nursing drug handbook 2010.* St. Louis, MO: Saunders Elsevier.

Homoud, M. K. (2008). *Introduction to antiarrhythmic agents.* Retrieved October 25, 2012, from http://ocw.tufts.edu/data/50/636944.pdf

Idioventricular rhythm and accelerated ventricular rhythm. Retrieved October 25, 2012, from www.cardionursing.com/pdfs/ch5.pdf

Junctional dysrhythmias. Retrieved October 21, 2012, from www.nursing.unboundmedicine.com/nursingcentral/ub/pview/.../JunctionalDysrhythmias

Junctional rhythm. Retrieved October 21, 2012, from www.equimedcorp .com/rhythms/topic/36/

Kulick, D. L., Lee, D., & Shiel, Jr., W. C. (2009, October). *Premature ventricular contractions (PVCs).* Retrieved October 26, 2012, from www.medicinenet.com/script/main/art.asp?articlekey=1946& pf=3&page=2

Landrum, M. A. (2012). *Fast facts for the critical care nurse: Critical care nursing in a nutshell.* New York, NY: Springer Publishing Company.

Lesson 3a: A cellular perspective: Electrophysiology of the heart. Retrieved November 7, 2012, from www.nuclearcardiologyseminars .net/electrophysiology.htm

Lesson 3b: The cardiac cycle and the conduction system. Retrieved November 7, 2012, from www.nuclearcardiologyseminars.net/ conduction.htm

Marill, K. A., Kazzi, A. A., Khalil, M. K., & Bright, A. A. (2011, June). *Ventricular fibrillation in emergency medicine.* Retrieved October 26, 2012, from www.emedicine.medscape.com/article/ 760832-overview

Marill, K. A., Kazzi, A. A., Khalil, M. K., & Bright, A. A. (2011, June). *Ventricular fibrillation in emergency medicine clinical presentation.* Retrieved October 26, 2012, from www.emedicine.medscape .com/article/760832-clinical

Mayo Clinic Staff. (2012, April). *Bundle branch block.* Retrieved November 1, 2012, from www.mayoclinic.com/health/bundle-branch-block?DS00693?METHOD=print&DSECTION=all

Pezeshkian, N. G., & Yang, Y. (2012, October). *Accelerated idioventricular rhythm.* Retrieved October 26, 2012, from www .emedicine.medscape.com/article/150074-overview

Pezeshkian, N. G., & Yang, Y. (2012, October). *Accelerated idioventricular rhythm clinical presentation.* Retrieved October 26, 2012, from www.emedicine.medscape.com/article/150074-clinical

Pezeshkian, N. G., & Yang, Y. (2012, October). *Accelerated idioventricular rhythm medication.* Retrieved October 26, 2012, from www.emedicine.medscape.com/article/150074-medication

Pezeshkian, N. G., & Yang, Y. (2012, October). *Accelerated idioventricular rhythm treatment & management.* Retrieved October 26, 2012, from www.emedicine.medscape.com/article/150074-treatment

Rosenthal, L., Borczuk, P., Chandrakantan, A., Greenberg, M. L., Kocheril, A. G., Lober, W., et al. (2012, October). *Atrial fibrillation treatment & management.* Retrieved October 21, 2012, from www.emedicine.medscape.com/article/151066-treatment#aw2aa b6b6b3

Rosenthal, L., & Ennis, C. A. (2011, November). *Atrial flutter.* Retrieved October 21, 2012, from "www.emedicine.medscape .com/article/151210-overview#a0104

Sovari, A. A., Gaeta, T. J., Kocheril, A. G., & Levine, M. D. (2011, September). *Second-degree atrioventricular block.* Retrieved October 28, 2012, from www.emedicine.medscape.com/ article/161919-overview#aw2aab6b2b3

Sovari, A. A., Gaeta, T. J., Kocheril, A. G., & Levine, M. D. (2011, September). *Second-degree atrioventricular block treatment & Management.* Retrieved October 28, 2012, from www.emedicine .medscape.com/article/161919-treatment

Springhill Medical Center. (2012). *Basic EKG rhythm identification.* Mobile, AL: Author.

Tandon, N., Hemphill, R. R., Huott, M. A., & Reddy, P. C. (2011, March). *Multifocal atrial tachycardia: Overview of multifocal atrial tachycardia.* Retrieved October 21, 2012, from www.emedicine .medscape.com/article/155825-overiew#showall

Index

Printed in the United States
By Bookmasters